AUTISM

AN ANCIENT FOE BECOMES
A MODERN SCOURGE–
THE RETURN OF A STEALTH BACTERIA

LAWRENCE BROXMEYER, MD

ISBN: 1478101261
ISBN-13: 9781478101260
Library of Congress Control Number: 2012911271
CreateSpace, North Charleston, SC

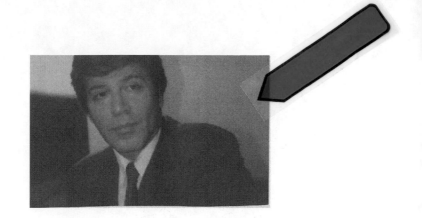

Lawrence Broxmeyer, MD, is a Pennsylvania internist and medical researcher. He was on staff at New York affiliate hospitals of SUNY Downstate, Cornell University, and New York University for approximately fourteen years. In conjunction with colleagues in San Francisco and at the University of Nebraska, he first pursued, as lead author and originator, a novel technique to kill AIDS mycobacteria and tuberculosis, producing outstanding results (see *Journal of Infectious Diseases* 186, no. 8 (October 15, 2002): 1155–60). Recently he contributed a chapter regarding these findings to Sleator and Hill's textbook *Pathobiotechnology*, published by Landes Bioscience. In addition, Broxmeyer has written many peer-reviewed articles, available on PubMed of the US Library of Medicine, National Institutes of Health, at: http://www.ncbi.nlm.nih.gov/pubmed?term=broxmeyer%20L. Broxmeyer's research covers the most challenging medical problems of our times, including AIDS, Alzheimer's disease, and now autism.

TABLE OF CONTENTS

1. INTRODUCTION

Writing in *Microbiology Today* in 2000, the UK's Dr.
Milton Wainwright, senior lecturer in Microbiology
at the Department of Molecular Biology and Biotechnology,
University of Sheffield, had a point.

University libraries all over the world are full of old scientific journals and books, left unread to gather dust. They
are ignored, said Wainwright, largely because most scientists and doctors think that anything that is more than, say,
10 years old is not worth bothering with. "Here, however,
offered Wainwright, "I want to suggest that these journals
represent a huge resource of untapped knowledge, a view
substantiated by numerous examples of where discoveries
turn out to be independent rediscoveries."

Of all the forgotten papers, stressed Wainwright, those relating to the cause or etiology of a disease are likely to be the most important.

Wainwright goes into the reasons for important old literature being ignored. Perhaps the study was singular in its material and may have just been overlooked. Or discoveries may have been dismissed because of the opposition from a single influential person. "The minor unwritten law of science", said Dr. Wainwright, "that 'one negative result (or a few) often outweighs many positives' often operates. The 'but everyone knows it is wrong' response is often used by people who have not even read the relevant literature."

The thesis of this manuscript ties evidence, old and new, that autism and childhood schizophrenia are indeed linked historically and scientifically; as are, schizophrenia and tuberculosis. From that point, it is merely a logical progression that if schizophrenia and tuberculosis are linked, it is quite possible, indeed conceivable, that autism and tuberculosis are as well. This paper makes the case for and cites papers pertaining to that causal relationship.

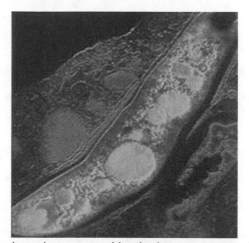

Figure 1: Tuberculosis, caused by the bacterium *Mycobacterium tuberculosis*, infects an estimated one third of the world's population.

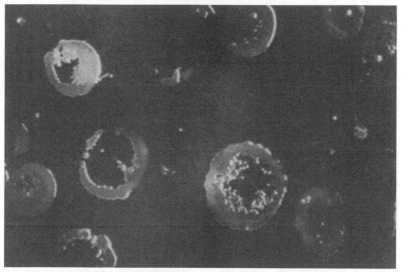

Figure 2. One of the STEALTH forms of "cell-wall deficient" atypical tuberculosis colonies that grew from the brain of a child who expired from the disease. Such forms of tuberculosis are extremely difficult to detect and require special stains and culture media not used routinely in today's laboratories. [From Korsak T., *Acta Tuberc. Pneumol. Belg., 66:445-469 1975*].

Autism can be defined as either (1.) A mental condition, present from early childhood, characterized by great difficulty in communicating and forming relationships with other people and in using language and abstract concepts, or, (2.) A mental condition in which fantasy dominates over reality, as a symptom of schizophrenia and other disorders.

The consensus that autism is caused by an intrauterine infection has been growing, bolstered by Patterson's (2007) and Fatemi's (2009) studies. John Langdon Down, a subset of whose developmentally disabled children were autistic, saw this infection "for the most part" as having its source in parental tuberculosis (TB), a disease that, according to the World Health Organization, presently infects over one-third of the world's inhabitants. Globally, at least one person is infected with TB per second, and someone dies of TB every ten seconds. Tuberculosis kills two to three million people each year, more than any other infectious disease in the world today. It would take such a disease to correlate with the growing incidence and prevalence of autism presently among us.

"John Langdon Down, a subset of whose developmentally disabled children were autistic, saw this infection "for the most part" as

having its source in parental tuberculosis (TB), a disease that, according to the World Health Organization, presently infects over one-third of the world's inhabitants."

The US National Institutes of Health reports that Indiana University has a clinical trial using the antitubercular drug Seromycin (cycloserine) for autism. A poor choice, Seromycin was never a first-line drug against TB, in large part because of its mind-bending side effects. The autistic child first presented in Leo Kanner's original study had to attend a tuberculosis "preventorium." Among the other mental sequella that the TB epidemic raging both in Kanner's time and today could cause was what Subramanian cited as "a withdrawal from social interaction." Yet Kanner studiously ignores the possible connection.

"Until almost 1980 autism was called childhood schizophrenia, and the link between autism and schizophrenia was thought undeniable."

Until almost 1980, autism was called childhood schizo-phrenia, and the link between autism and schizophrenia was thought undeniable. By 2010, Dr. Annemie Ploeger still saw schizophrenia and autism as probably sharing a common origin, both with physical abnormalities that form during the first month of pregnancy. And Rzhetsky(2007), using a proof-of-concept biostatistical analysis of one and a half million patient records, found significant genetic overlap in humans with autism, schizophrenia,.......... and tuberculosis.

Not only is tuberculosis the most common cause of infec-tious death in children and their childbearing mothers, but it is extremely neurotropic and remains, worldwide, the most common type of central nervous system infection, particu-larly among children. Twenty to 25 percent of these young victims can manifest mental retardation as well as other anomalies often associated with the neurodevelopmental disorders of the autistic spectrum.

Although the brain and spinal cord are considered immune-privileged organs in that they are separated from the rest of the body via the blood-brain barrier, Calmette's studies at Institut Pasteur showed that viral forms of cell-wall-compromised tuberculosis (cell-wall-deficient forms) had little problem reach-ing vulnerable nervous tissue in the brain.

"Globally, at least one person is infected with TB per second, and someone dies of TB every ten seconds. Tuberculosis kills two to three million people each year, more than any other infectious disease in the world today."

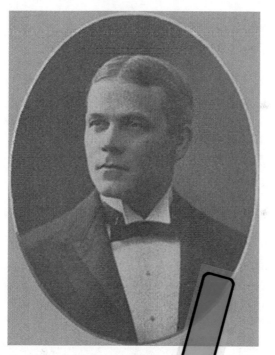

Figure 3. Dr Aldred Scott WARTHIN, MD (1866-1931) Head of Pathology at the University of Michigan, Ann Arbor. Warthin saw that fetal tissues were relatively immune to the action of the tubercle bacillus. Yet such infection was transmitted through the placenta, even in mothers without signs of infection to her fetus. This created

a situation where a truly latent tuberculosis was both possible and probable, with tissue changes developing some time after birth, and at a rate "much more frequently than is generally supposed."

Since the turn of the twentieth century, there have been adequate warnings regarding both the extent of maternal-fetal transmission of tuberculosis and its implications in the etiology of childhood schizophrenia. Warnings from many sources. It wasn't only from Calmette voicing them from Pasteur. Ann Arbor pathologist Warthin, in an article appearing in the *Journal of Infectious Diseases*, said that it was highly probable that when a woman with silent foci of tuberculosis in her body and with no symptoms whatsoever became pregnant, she could experience reactivation of her disease. That, in turn, could transmit pregnancy-reactivated, blood-borne tuberculous bacilli to her child while it was still in her uterus. Nor, he emphasized, was this either rare or uncommon. Physician F. Parkes Weber, in an article appearing in the *British Journal of Children's Diseases*, agreed, adding that in those cases in which the disease attacked fetal tissue, it apparently did not occur before the fourth month of pregnancy.

"Rzhetsky(2007), using a proof-of-concept biostatistical analysis of one and a half million patient

records, found significant genetic overlap in humans with autism, schizophrenia,.........and tuberculosis."

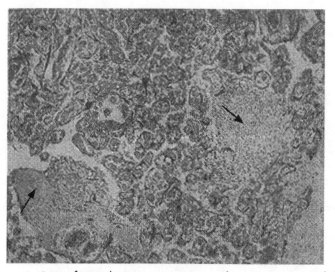

Figure 4. One of Warthin's tissue mounts. The transmission of the tubercle bacilli to the fetus from a mother with unrecognized, latent tuberculosis with no maternal symptoms. Two miliary tubercles (see arrows) have formed in the placenta, brought there through the maternal bloodstream [A.S. Warthin, MD, Ph.D. "Miliary Tuberculosis of The Placenta" *JAMA* Vol LXI, No. 22 1951-52].

Warthin saw silent asymptomatic tuberculosis during pregnancy as a danger not only to the mother but a "very grave danger" to her fetus. A professor of pathology and director of the pathology lab at the University of Michigan, Warthin had once taught Rous, and now relentlessly followed cases of maternal TB being transmitted through the placenta. He mentions that such pregnancy-activated tubercle bacilli could, in certain cases, pass through the placenta into fetal circulation— initially without even causing changes to either placental structure or fetal tissue. In such cases, it could only be found in fetal blood. Warthin's findings, together with Calmette's findings, present the picture of a true stealth pathogen that often left few fingerprints in its progression. Calmette clarified the covert nature of the disease, confirming that TB's attack form going through the virtual filters of the placenta into fetal blood consisted mainly of viral, filter-passing forms of tuberculosis, something that Nobel nominee Lida Mattman for decades called the preferred form of tuberculosis. Such forms, Mattman stressed, required special stains and cultures for detection that are not routinely used in current US laboratories.

By 1997, Adhikari and Pillay saw tuberculosis in the newborn as an emerging problem, again, even in mothers with subclinical, asymptomatic maternal TB. Norris, whose textbook is routinely used in medical schools, again points out that pregnancy-activated latent tuberculosis could lead to febrile, bacteremic, blood-borne episodes. Just as importantly, Harrison reminds us that not only is tuberculosis an important cause of fever of unknown origin (FUO), but tuberculosis outside the lungs, as in its blood-bearing stage, is *the* most frequent cause of FUO, an issue that Zerbo's 2012 UC Davis study does not specifically address. Zerbo et al., while ruling out influenza, did show that fever during pregnancy more than doubles the risk of autism or developmental delay in children. Coury, in response, urged caution regarding the fever-autism link, saying, "It is an association, and doesn't mean that maternal fever causes autism, just that we see these two occurring more frequently than other things." Perhaps the fever itself does not cause autism, but that does not mean that the fever's underlying cause, were it an infection, didn't.

By 1999, Pillet reviewed the difficulties in early diagnosis of neonatal tuberculosis, finding it again grossly underestimated. In fact so difficult is cerebral tuberculosis to diagnose in infants that Rock *et al*, in an April 2008 issue of *Clinical Microbiology Reviews*, mentions that some pediatric experts recommend that all children under 12 months of age should have a lumbar puncture due to both their susceptibility to cerebral tuberculosis and the difficulty in clinically evaluating infants with it. This is controversial, however the difficulty in clinical evaluation mentioned is not.

By 2003, Gourion and others reported on how neonatal cerebral tuberculosis had evolved into a member of the autistic spectrum of disorders, namely Asperger's syndrome. More importantly, a cross-comparison between neuropathology and imaging studies done on TB menin-goencephalitis (Hosoglu 1998 and Ozates 2000) and those from the autistic spectrum (Murphy 2002), (Haznedar 1993), and (Happe 1996)seemed to match. Indeed, Schoeman's study implied that tuberculosis and its neonatal brain lesions were behind all neurodevelopmental disorders, including the autistic spectrum.

Many hypotheses regarding what causes autism have been and will continue to be put forth, just as there was in the case of tuberculosis, which was blamed on heredity, chemicals, and even on how one maintained his or her posture. But there was only one definitive answer in the case of tuberculosis, just as there will be, in the future, for autism.

L.B

"Indeed, Schoeman's study implied that tuberculosis and its neonatal brain lesions were behind all neurodevelopmental disorders, including the autistic spectrum."

KEYWORDS: autism, autistic spectrum, Asperger's syndrome, developmental disorders, schizophrenia, childhood schizophrenia,   mycobacterial infection, *Mycobacterium tuberculosis*, history of autism, cell-wall-deficient mycobacteria, Leo Kanner, Down syndrome, John Langdon Down, tuberculosis.

2. CALIFORNIA DEPARTMENT OF DEVELOPMENTAL SERVICES, SACRAMENTO, 1999

California, in 1999, had been on high alert for some time. Level-one autism, without any of its "spectrum," went from almost five thousand cases in late summer 1993 to an estimated 20,377 cases by December 2002. As California's Department of Developmental Services stood by incredulously, it witnessed a tripling of California's autism rate, and all but 15 percent of cases were in children.

California wasn't alone. But its autism rates had become the fastest growing group in that state's developmental disability system, and a number of Bay Area school districts were forced to fill entire classes with youths with different forms of autism.

But even in the midst of California's mini-epidemic, its Santa Clara County seemed particularly singled out. The Department of Social Services Aid, brokered by the San Andreas Regional Center, staggered to its breaking point, and its forecast for autism in Santa Clara wasn't good.

What was behind this epidemic? A major clue, overlooked from a critical standpoint, was contained in the time line of the department's own 1999 autism report, which concluded that the disease had increased dramatically between 1987 and 1998.

What had happened in California in and around 1987 that could have sown the surplus of autism that California now reaped?

3. DIVISION OF COMMUNICABLE DISEASES, SACRAMENTO, CALIFORNIA, 1999

While autism exploded in California, there was also, beginning in 1987, a major spike in the number of tuberculosis cases reported by the Tuberculosis Control Branch of California's Division of Communicable Disease. There, division head Dr. Sarah Royce proclaimed a TB epidemic in California. The epidemic peaked in 1992, had the same male preponderance as autism, and took off at precisely the same moment in time.

California's TB epidemic might have already peaked well before 1999, but this didn't stop it from continuing to contribute the greatest number of cases to the nation's total tuberculosis morbidity.[1] But, as with autism, the problem was worldwide, and even the World Health Organization, traditionally slow to react, had declared a global tuberculosis emergency six years earlier,[2] a warning that has been in existence ever since.

Among children, brain-seeking central nervous system tuberculosis is common in a disease that kills more children each year than any other, with the potential to cause in survivors, among other things in its devastating wake, a withdrawal from social interaction.[3]

It had to be more than a coincidence, therefore, that since the 1980s, California experienced a dramatic increase in the number of children diagnosed with autism as well.[4]

1. Ussery, X.T., Valway, S.E., McKenna, M., et al. Epidemiology of Tuberculosis among Children in the United States. *Pediatric Infectious Disease Journal*, 15 (1996): 697–704.

2. Dolin, P.J., Raviglione, M.C., and Kochi, A. "Global Tuberculosis Incidence and Mortality during 1990–2000. *Bull of the World Health Organization*, 72 (1994): 213–20.

3. Subramanian, P. Extrapulmonary Tuberculosis. In *Walsh & Hoyt's Clinical Neuro-Opthalmology*, Vol. 3.

Edited by Neil R. Miller, MD and Nancy Newman, MD. [Philadelphia]: Lippincott, Williams & Wilkins, 2005, 2690.

4. California Department of Developmental Services. *Autistic Spectrum Disorders Changes in the California Caseload: An Update: 1999 through 2002.* Sacramento, April 3, 2004.

4. SANTA CLARA COUNTY CALIFORNIA, MARCH 2006

If California was experiencing autistic tremors, then surely its Santa Clara County was at the epicenter. By 2006, Santa Clara had some of the highest rates for autism in the entire country. And although this was for unknown reasons, again the question became, why Santa Clara? And the answer pointed in a similar direction. By 2002, it had become apparent that TB was on the rise in Santa Clara, and, by 2006, that county had the highest number of new TB cases in California.

Santa Clara's Health Department sounded the alarm. Santa Clara now knew that it had two problems on its hands. Its medically trained psychiatrists, personnel and statisticians just never stopped to think that the two problems might be related.

"Santa Clara's Health Department sounded the alarm. Santa Clara now knew that it had two problems on its hands."

5. CENTERS FOR DISEASE CONTROL AND PREVENTION, ATLANTA, GEORGIA, SEPTEMBER 2008

Time passed. More information came to in.

In September 2008, the Centers for Disease Control and Prevention published a study by lead author, pediatrician, and researcher Laura J. Christie of the California Department of Public Health entitled "Diagnostic Challenges of Central Nervous System Tuberculosis." Christie and colleagues identified twenty cases of unexplained encephalitis referred to the California Encephalitis Project that were indeed tubercular.[1] The team importantly began with the significant statement that "Tuberculosis (TB) of the central nervous system (CNS)" as thought of by physicians, "is classically described as meningitis. However, altered mental status, including encephalitis is within the spectrum of clinical manifestations."

Indeed, according to Seth and Kabra, central nervous system tuberculosis in children can also include tuberculous vasculopathy (infection of cerebral blood vessels), small tubercular masses called tuberculomas or TB abscesses.[2]

In most of the twenty cases, the California Encephalitis Project cultured out tuberculous, the same tuberculosis considered the least likely cause for encephalitis. Yet there it was. But, as Christie pointed out, as little as 25 percent of patients with a diagnosis of CNS TB actually culture out TB, which was a criteria for this particular study. That means that only 1/4th of possible cases were being diagnosed. And even the most sophisticated diagnostic lab tests proved not helpful in further probing the culture proven cases. This leads us to believe that the 75 percent that were diagnosed as possible CNS TB in the clinics, but had negative cultures would probably also not have been also not diagnostically picked up with the same sophisticated tests.

"The team importantly began with the significant statement that "Tuberculosis (TB) of the central

nervous system (CNS)" as thought of by physicians, "is classically described as meningitis. However, altered mental status, including encephalitis is within the spectrum of clinical manifestations."

1. Christie, L. J., Loeffler, A. M., Honamand, S., Flood, J. M., Baxter, R., Jacobson, S., Alexander, R., and Glaser, C.A. "Diagnostic Challenges of Central Nervous System Tuberculosis." *Emerg Infec Dis.*, 14, no. 9 (September 2008): 1473–75.

2. Seth, V., and Kabra, S. K. *Essentials of Tuberculosis in Children.* [Delhi]: Jaypee Brothers, 2006.

6. OFFICE OF THE MEDICAL SUPERINTENDENT, EARLSWOOD ASYLUM FOR IDIOTS, SURREY ENGLAND, 1887

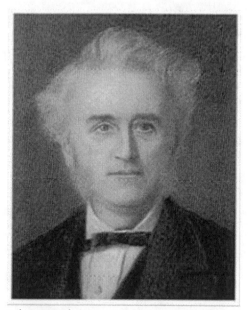

Figure 5. Dr. John Langdon Down [18 November 1828 – 7 October 1896]. According to George T. Capsone, M.D., Down's original report attributed Down syndrome to maternal tuberculosis.

It was in the teachings of John Langdon Down, some of whose "mentally retarded" children were autistic, that Leo Kanner really found his autism.

Down, one of the outstanding medical scholars of his day, was certain to gain entrance into the prominent London Hospital when he decided instead to pursue an avenue few would entertain, as superintendent of the Earlswood Asylum for Idiots in Surrey. But for Down, it was preordained. At the age of eighteen, he had what might be described as a transformative experience. A heavy summer storm drove his family to take shelter in a cottage. Down wrote: "I was brought into contact with a feeble minded girl, who waited on our party and for whom the question haunted me—could nothing for her be done? I had then not entered on a medical student's career but ever and anon…the remembrance of that hapless girl presented itself to me and I longed to do something for her kind."[1]

"It was in the teachings of John Langdon Down, some of whose "mentally retarded" children were autistic, that Leo Kanner really found his autism."

Down, therefore, became a doctor for reasons that were the purist of them all, and he soon excelled and became the head of his class. His pursuits were brought to a temporary halt when he acquired tuberculosis, which sent him back to his family's home in Torpoint. Gradually, he recovered. Down then went through an obstetrics residency before obtaining his MD to assume the position of head of the Earlswood Asylum. He was now quite knowledgeable about pregnancy, the complications and diseases of pregnancy, and neonates. In addition, his surgical skills allow him to do autopsies, during which he contributes much to expand knowledge of conditions of the brain such as cerebral palsy as well as probe into what had killed the children in his institution that died from Down syndrome.

In his Lettsonian Lectures, Down follows the psychiatric nomenclature of his time and classifies his most severe cases of mental retardation in the young under the category of "idiocy."[2] Like Kanner, he specifies that some of his mentally retarded children had exceptional intellect in specific areas, such as memorization, music, or mathematics. In fact, a noticeable subset of the autistic children that Down treated did not appear physically to even have mental retardation.

Gillberg and Coleman relate that quite a number of reports of individuals with Down syndrome also meet the criteria for autism.[3]

By 1867, John Langdon Down had appeared in the *Lancet*, linking childhood mental illness with tuberculosis.[4] To Down, in fact, children who inherited Down syndrome "for the most part, arose from tuberculosis in the parents" and not genetics.[5] Capone mentions that Down's original report attributed the condition to maternal tuberculosis.[6] As a result of such tuberculosis from conception or soon thereafter, and nothing else, such children's life expectancy would be shortened, as the same tuberculous infection would lead to their early demise.

"Dr. George T. Capone mentions that Down's original report attributed the condition to maternal tuberculosis."

The only thing really wrong with John Langdon Down's theory was that it was way ahead of its time.

He knew that tuberculosis was, as it still is, the most common cause of death from a single infectious agent in children,[7] now killing upwards of 250,000 children each year,[8] yet exceedingly difficult to diagnose.[9] He also knew that TB was the single leading cause of death among women of reproductive age, between fifteen and forty-four, one million of whom presently die, according to the World Health Organization, each year.[10]

Brain and central nervous system tuberculosis account for 20 to 45 percent of all types of tuberculosis among children, much higher than its rate of 2.9 to 5.9 percent for all adult tuberculosis.[11] In fact, tuberculosis of the nervous system has consistently been the second most common form of TB outside of the lung in the very young.

And of those infants and children who did survive, nearly 20 to 25 percent manifested mental retardation and mental disorders[12]—serious and long-term behavioral disturbances,[13] seizures,[14] and motor (movement) handicaps in addition to the various other anomalies associated with the autistic spectrum and what Down called "neurodevelopmental" behavior problems.

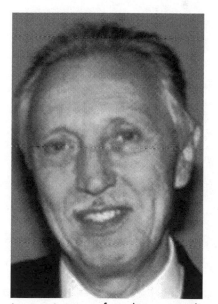

Figure 6. Dr. Jérome Lejeume found an extra chromosome on Chromosome 21 in Down Syndrome. However, to this day nobody has

come up with the actual cause for this genetic abnormality and studies such as Shy-Ching Lo's 2004 study at the Armed Forces Institute of Pathology have since shown that such karyotypic changes can result from infection itself.

"..when Lejeune faced McGill geneticists at a Montreal Congress of Genetics, announcing that he had located an extra chromosome in the karyotype of Down syndrome patients and showed it to them, he was received with interest but skepticism.... considerable skepticism."

Today, Down is considered wrong for saying that Down syndrome was caused by parental tuberculosis and rather that it is a "genetic" abnormality, an extra chromosome on Chromosome 21 called trisomy. But was Down really wrong? To this day, no one has come up with the actual cause for this genetic abnormality. This was probably why the discoverer of the extra chromosome, Frenchman Jérome Lejeune, hesitated to publish results that were otherwise clear-cut. And when Lejeune faced McGill geneticists at a

Montreal Congress of Genetics, announcing that he had located an extra chromosome in the karyotype of Down syndrome patients and showed it to them, he was received with interest but skepticism.... considerable skepticism.

Since, Warthin,[15] Rao,[16] Lakimenko,[17] and Golubchick[18] have all revealed how tuberculosis itself can cause chromosomal change reminiscent of those found in Lejeune's trisomy. Warthin showed tuberculosis's early penetration right into the corpus luteum itself , in which 90 percent of Down syndrome's abnormal meiotic chromosomal splitting occurs. Rao also found that the tubercle bacillus is capable of inducing such chromosomal changes as result in Down syndrome's nondisjunction of the human egg. And Lakimenko and Golubchick independently proved just how devastating TB could be to the chromosomal apparatus of cell cultures of the human amnion, in not one, but two independent studies. Each showed an increase in pathological mitoses, arrest of cell division in metaphase, and the actual appearance of chromosomal adhesions absent in control cultures. Indeed, Lakimenko and Golubchick demonstrated that early tubercular involvement was not only destructive against chromosomes but the very spindles that separated them. Total ovarian destruction occurs in 3 percent of women with pelvic tuberculosis,[19] again the site where Down syndrome's and autism's chromosomal abnormalities usually occur.

For his *Lancet* study, Down submits one hundred post mortem records of children who had passed away at his institution. He had found no fewer than 62 percent of these children to have tubercular deposits in their bodies. For some unknown reason, boys had more than twice the incidence of tubercles in their organs as did girls, a finding that concurred with the male predominance he later notes in childhood mental disease in general. Such male preponderance is today not only documented in Down syndrome but in autism as well. Tuberculosis might be more frequently transmitted by the mother than the father, but it was the male offspring who were more tubercular. Caldecott, in a 1909 *British Medical Journal* article, noted that Down showed that the children in his study rarely lived beyond twenty years as a consequence of brain and nervous system disease, and that they died of...... tuberculosis.[20]

1. Down, J. Langdon. Address Christian Union, June 27, 1879.
2. Down, J. L. *On Some of the Mental Affectations of Childhood and Youth. The Lettsonian Lectures.* London: J&A Churchill, 1887.
3. Gillberg, C., and Coleman, M. The Biology of the Autistic Syndromes, in *Clinics in Developmental Medicine*, No. 153/4 3rd Edition Mac Keith Press 2000, 140.

4. Down, J. L. On Idiocy and Its Relation to Tuberculosis *The Lancet*, 2 (1867).
5. Down, J.L.H. Observations on an Ethnic Classification of Idiots. *Lond Hosp Clin Lect*, Rep 3 (1866): 259–62.
6. Capone, G. T. Down Syndrome: Advances in Molecular Biology and the Neurosciences, *Developmental and Behavioral Pediatrics*, 22, no. 1 (February 2001): 40-59.
7. Walia, R., and Hoskyns, W. Tuberculous Meningitis in Children: Problem to Be Addressed Effectively with Thorough Contact Tracing *Eur J Pediatr.*, 159, no. 7 (July 2000): 535–38.
8. Titone, L., and Romano, A. Epidemiology of Paediatric Tuberculosis Today Infez Med, 11, no. 3 (September 2003): 127–32.
9. Mahadevan, B., and Mahadevan, S. Tuberculin Reactivity in Tuberculosis Meningitis *Indian J. Pediatr.*, 72, no. 3 (March 2005): 213–15.
10. World Health Organization. *TB Is Single Biggest Killer of Young Women*. Press Release, no. 40. Geneva, Switzerland: World Health Organization, May 26, 1998.
11. Molavi, A., and Lefrock, J.L. Tuberculous Meningitis. *Med Clin North Am*, 69 (1985): 315–31.
12. Garg, P.K. Tuberculosis of the Central Nervous System. *Post grad Med J*, 75 (1999): 133–40.

13. Schoeman, J.F., and Springer, P. Adjunctive Thalidomide Therapy for Childhood Tuberculous Meningitis: Results of a Randomized Study. *J. Child Neurol*, 19, no. 4 (April 2004): 250–57.

14. Takamatsu, I. The Current Situation and Treatment of Childhood Tuberculosis *Kekkaku*, 74, no. 4 (April 1999): 365–75.

15. Warthin, A. S., and Cowie, D. M. A Contribution in the Casuistry of Placental and Congenital Tuberculosis. *Journ. Inf. Dis.*, 1 (1904): 140.

16. Rao, V. V., Gupta, E. V., and Thomas, I. M. Chromosome Damage in Untreated Tuberculosis Patients. *Tubercle.*, 71, no. 3 (September 1990): 169–72.

17. Lakimenko, L. N. Changes in the Mitotic Regime of a Cell Culture under the Influence of Sensitins. *Biull Eksp Biol Med.*, 81, no. 2 (February 1976): 237–39.

18. Golubchik, I. S., Lakimenko, L. N., and Lazovskaia, A. L. Effect of Tuberculin on the Mitotic Regime in Cell Cultures *Biull Eksp Biol Med.*, 73, no. 5 (May 1972): 105–7.

19. Nogales-Ortiz, F., and Tarancon, I. The Pathology of Female Genital Tuberculosis. *Obstet. Gynecol.*, 53 (1979): 422-428

20. Caldecott, H. Discussion of Paper by Shuttleworth GE: Mongolian Imbecility. *British Medical Journal*, 2 (1909): 661–65.

7. DEPARTMENT OF PSYCHIATRY, BURGHOLZLI HOSPITAL, ZURICH, SWITZERLAND, 1930

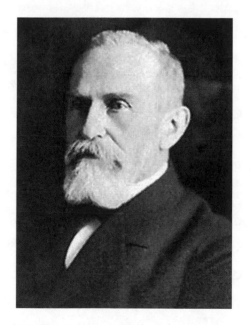

Figure 7. Paul Eugen Bleuler Born April 30, 1857 - Died July 15,1939 (aged 82) Zollikon, Switzerland He coined the word *schizophrenia*. In

1908 Bleuler described the main symptoms of
schizophrenia as 4 A's: flattened *Affect*, *Autism*,
impaired *Association* of ideas and *Ambivalence*.

The word *autism* first appeared in English in the April 1913 issue of the *American Journal of Insanity*,[1] heralded at an address that Swiss psychiatrist Paul Eugen Bleuler delivered for the opening of Johns Hopkins University's Henry Phipps Psychiatric Clinic.

Bleuler used the word autism, Greek for "self," to describe the difficulty that people with schizophrenia experience connecting with other people, and, in certain cases, withdrawing into their own world and showing self-centered thought. But to Bleuler, schizophrenia, and thereby autism, still came from an organic cause such as infection, and, as such, was sometimes curable. Until about 1980, autism and schizophrenia were considered basically one and the same. To that point, Bleuler's definition holds.

Bleuler also uses *autistic* to describe doctors who are not attached to scientific reality, wont to build on what Bleuler calls "autistic ways"—that is, through methods in no way supported by scientific evidence, an event more and more in evidence as psychiatrists moved away from tissue-based outcomes into the realm of subjective behavior labeling. The history of autism would see many such individuals.

"Bleuler used the word autism, Greek for "self," to describe the difficulty that people with schizophrenia experience connecting with other people, and, in certain cases, withdrawing into their own world and showing self-centered thought." ·

1. Bleuler, E. Autistic Thinking. *American Journal of Insanity*, 69, no. 5 (April 1913): 873.

8. CHILD PSYCHIATRY SERVICE, JOHNS HOPKINS UNIVERSITY HOSPITAL, PEDIATRIC DIVISION, BALTIMORE, 1933

Internal-medicine-trained Leo Kanner teaches himself the basics of child psychiatry and, at the instigation of Adolph Meyer, joins the Henry Phipps Psychiatric Clinic at John Hopkins Hospital in Baltimore.

By 1903, Henry Phipps, wealthy partner of Andrew Carnegie, sought charitable outlets for his wealth. He then joined Lawrence F. Flick, a doctor with a vision, to open a center solely dedicated to the study, treatment, and prevention of tuberculosis, hands down the number-one infectious killer in the United States.

Not until May 1908 did Philadelphia steel magnate Phipps get around to visiting Johns Hopkins's tuberculosis division, which he had funded. At that point Phipps turns to ask John Hopkins's dean and legendary pathologist William Henry Welch if he needed help sponsoring other projects at the Hospital. Welch answers Phipps by handing him a copy of A Mind That Found Itself, an agonizing assessment of mental asylums written by Clifford W. Beers and published with the help of Swiss-born pathologist Adolph Meyer.[1] Within a month, Phipps agrees to donate $1.5 million to fund a psychiatric clinic for the Johns Hopkins Department of Psychiatry. By 1912, the Henry Phipps Psychiatric Service at Johns Hopkins Hospital provides the first in-patient psychiatric facility in the United States for the mentally ill.

Welch likes Meyer.

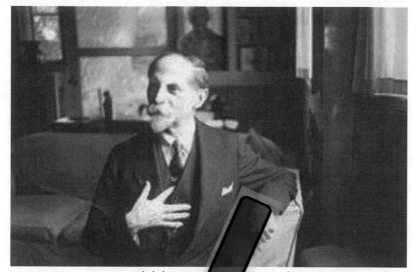

Figure 8. Dr. Adolph Meyer. Born September 13, 1866 Niederwenigen - Died March 17, 1950 (age 83) Baltimore. Head of Johns Hopkin's psychiatry. One of the most influential figures in American psychiatry in the first half of the Twentieth Century. Under Meyer's auspices and direction the first academic department of child psychiatry in the world was founded by Leo Kanner in 1930.

Meyer, although unable to secure an appointment from his alma mater, the University of Zurich, is, like Welch, a pathologist—a neuropathologist to be exact. Also Welch takes to him because Meyer initially seems to reject Freud as the be-all and end-all for psychiatry. And there is another level of understanding: Meyer and Welch share the rapport of two superb medical networkers and politicians. Welch sees to it that Meyer becomes the head of psychiatry at Johns Hopkins.

But it is the very same second-rate, vague, "psycho-biological" views that characterize Meyer's psychiatric approach that will prove in the end to be disappointing. Designed to be all things to all people, Meyer's psychobiology assesses mental patients' physical and psychosocial problems concomitantly, but turns out to be all things to no one. Meyer is much more oriented towards taking extensive histories of his patients; getting all the "facts", then in rooting out the pathology behind mental illness on the autopsy table. Besides, the positions of Meyer and Freud closely resemble one another in that each insists heavily on the study of psychogenic factors in neurotic disorders. Welch, on the other hand, was committed to bringing the German model, which relied heavily on the lab, to US medicine. So with Meyer, Welch didn't precisely get what he thought he was getting.

Nevertheless, thanks to neurologist and pathologist Adolph Meyer, Leo Kanner becomes the first "child psychiatrist" at Johns Hopkins and, by default, in the United States. Meyer is bent on changing American psychiatry, and will dominate psychiatry from his Johns Hopkins chair during the first half of the twentieth century.

Meyer has long been interested in the psychiatric treatment of children, so he arranges with Johns Hopkins pediatrician Edwards Park for Kanner to become a liaison between pediatrics and psychiatry at the institution. This gives Kanner enhanced influence in reaching an audience of pediatricians who otherwise would have found little value in the psychiatric evaluation of children. Meyer has already decided that the psychosocial aspects of mental disease are more important than tissue diagnosis of brain pathology. He closes his laboratory, and instead prefers talking to his patients, taking extensive histories in the manner of Kraepelin and Sigmund Freud.

"Nevertheless, thanks to neurologist and pathologist Adolph Meyer, Leo Kanner becomes the first "child psychiatrist" at Johns Hopkins and, by default, in the United States".

1. Beers, C. W. *A Mind That Found Itself.* Pittsburgh, PA: University of Pittsburgh Press, 1981.

9. OFFICE OF NEUROLOGIST SIGMUND FREUD, VIENNA, AUSTRIA, 1883

Loudest of all is the cry: tuberculosis! Is it contagious? Is it acquired? Where does it come from? Is Master Koch of Berlin right in saying that he has discovered the bacillus responsible for it?[1]

Sigmund Freud, October 9, 1883

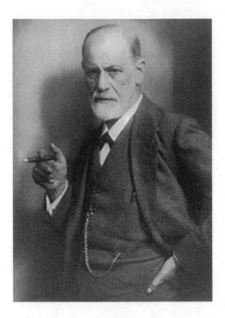

Figure 9. Sigmund Freud, 1921 [Born 6 May 1856 - Died 23 September 1939 (aged 83)] Sigmund Freud saw patients of whom he described the "satisfaction of the instincts is partially or totally withdrawn from the influence of other people.", a description that could fit present day concepts of autism. The influence of Freud's psychogenic hypothesis was not lost on Dr. Leo Kanner. In a 1960 interview, Kanner bluntly described parents of autistic children as "just happening to defrost enough to produce a child."

Long before Leo Kanner, Freud speculated that autism was an impairment in social functioning in which the satisfaction of instincts was, to one degree or another, withdrawn from the influence of other people. Freud's influence on psychology during the 1940s and 1950s is evident in the theories behind the cause of autism, including Leo Kanner's. Freudian psychologists suggested that children with autism were not given the proper love and attention they required in order to develop healthy interpersonal relationships. The theory remained popular through the early 1960s, and in certain pockets, still is.

Freud's prior neurophysiological interests leads him to the psychiatry clinic of famous brain anatomist and psychiatrist Theodor Meynert. Under Meynert, Freud proves unusually adept at diagnosing organic brain disorders, particularly the effects of localized injuries. But what he did not seem to pick up is Meynert's absolute belief that the root and cause of mental illness lie in the diseases and pathology in the human brain and central nervous system. Freud is unhappy with a career that might pursue such orthodoxy, as he expresses in a letter to his fiancée in 1884. Instead, he tells her, he is looking for "a lucky hit." That "lucky hit" would, of course, eventually turn out to be psychoanalysis and his talking cure.

"The first to mention tuberculosis-induced neuroses such as hysteria was Cardanus, who described a case cured in twenty days because it "merely involved the intellect." Thus, the first "talking

*cure" might have been on a
tuberculous patient well over two
hundred years before Freud."*

But even after he abandons Meynert's brain
approaches, Freud continues to admit that his wide-rang-
ing psychoanalytic theories would eventually need to be
rooted in the tissue neuroscience of Meynert. Otherwise,
he writes, it would only take "a few dozen years" to "blow
away" the "artificial structure of hypotheses" involved in
psychoanalysis.[2]

There are obvious holes In Freud's theories. But, for decades, nobody is picking them up. No one could deny the
tremendous impact his thoughts had on those working with
children with emotional problems. Nevertheless, Freud's theories at times seem to distort the treatment of serious mental
illnesses, among them the notion that bad mothering probably caused conditions such as schizophrenia. Not only did
this leave irrevocable guilt, in certain cases, on the families involved, but often on the patients themselves. Yet such
thoughts influenced a generation of thinkers. Kanner refers
to remnants of Freud in his "cold hearted moms," who he
finds often among his "autistic" children. In his book *Child
Psychiatry*, Kanner acknowledges Freud's merit more often
than not, although he later lashes out that Freud's influence

had gone too far, with many of Freud's followers insisting that his theories were just about infallible.

Leaving Meynert, Freud joins neurologist Charcot in Paris, who was working on the medical disorder "hysteria" — a wastebasket category that included depression and "conversion" disorders that produced pain with no obvious organic cause. It was in conversion hysteria that Charcot could sometimes, briefly, eliminate symptoms through hypnosis. Freud still felt that such hysteria had nothing to do with disease or brain pathology, which immediately put him at odds with most of the medical establishment of his day.

The first to mention tuberculosis-induced neuroses such as hysteria was Cardanus, who described a case cured in twenty days because it "merely involved the intellect."[3] Thus, the first "talking cure" might have been on a tuberculous patient well over two hundred years before Freud.

Once in private practice, Freud persists in using post-hypnotic suggestion to cure hysterical symptoms, to little avail. Finally, his great breakthrough comes not with one of his own patients, but when he utilizes the records of a patient who his friend and colleague Josef Breuer saw, "Anna O.", the first patient upon whom a "talking cure" was affected. Anna O. was Bertha Pappenheim, a twenty-one-year-old woman who developed a host of physical and mental problems while attending to her father, who died of tuberculosis. Some of her own symptoms included an intractable cough, severe headache, malaise, partial paralysis, and vision problems.......... were all thought by Freud to be "hysterical." Suffering from epilepsy, one of her arms was paralyzed as a result of complex seizures.

Based on all of these symptoms, even Breuer, in his chart notes, seriously considers that Anna O. has tuberculosis meningitis. Then, discovering that her paralyzed arm was the one that cradled her dying father, Breuer makes the leap that she was unconsciously immobilizing her arm as self-inflicted punishment because she inwardly blamed herself for her father's death. Breuer then tries to get her to "talk out" her repressed memories to affect a cathartic cure. Breuer's case proves pivotal by Freud's own admission.

It was the beginning of a "psychoanalysis" which Freud would embellish from that point on. Freud presses Breuer for joint publication of *Studies on Hysteria*, accomplished in 1895. But even in this book, the gulf between Breuer and Freud was obvious. Breuer was an internist, trained in internal medicine, so he looked for neurologic disease processes behind Anna O.'s hysteria. Freud, on the other hand, used a psychological point of reference. What unfolded In the case of Anna O. would prove to be medical misjudgments with lasting consequences.

As the years went on, it became obvious to others that Anna O.'s more noteworthy symptoms pointed toward specific, infectious brain pathology, typical of complex partial seizures, originating in the temporal lobe. German-born research psychologist Hans J. Eysenck[4] and others speculate that Anna O. wasn't suffering from hysteria or neurosis at all, but brain involvement from tuberculosis, a disease that caused the death of two of her siblings at the ages of two and eighteen and a disease that her mother had and that she was again exposed to from nursing her tubercular-ridden, dying father.

According to Thornton's more in-depth account, Anna O.'s father had a tubercular abscess just under the lining (or "pleura") of one lung, a frequent complication of tuberculosis, which was then highly prevalent in Vienna. Nursing him exposed her to constant contact. Moreover, in the midst of Breuer's talking therapy,[5] Anna O.'s father's lung abscess was surgically incised and drained at home, subjecting the young woman, who changed his dressings, to direct exposure to his tubercular bacilli. The virulence of the strain that exuded from the purulent drainage from her father's chest tube was best attested to by the fact that it would soon kill him. Thornton makes it crystal clear that Freud's account of Anna O. was totally deceptive and that there had been no "talking cure" or catharsis, something he believed Freud knew very well.

Eysenck, famed for his Eysenck Personality Scale, said that it was neither Breuer nor Freud who really cured Anna O. but repeated hospitalizations for tubercular symptoms that occurred subsequent to their psychoanalytic treatment. Eysenck had a good case, and H. F. Ellenberger agreed.[6] Tracking down actual chart records, Ellenberger notes that Anna O.'s condition actually got much worse during Breuer's treatment, to the point where she had to be treated in a TB sanitarium. Again, Freud was aware of all this, but his account still proclaimed Anna O.'s pristine talking cure. Breuer, not nearly so enamored with the treatment he himself had originated, broke with Freud. And Jung was the first to point out publicly that the alleged success of the treatment of Anna O. was anything but. Jung insisted that there was no cure at all in the sense with which it was originally presented. Again, he mentions that Anna O. was not suffering from a neurosis at all, but from the mental and physical changes of a tuberculous meningitis that she had somehow survived.

Even Freud's case study of "Dora," which established Freud's theories about lesbians and female hysterics, was not untainted by physical disease. Dora was Ida Bauer, born in Vienna in 1882 of Bohemian Jewish ancestry. Dora's father, Philip, died of tuberculosis in 1913, one year after her mother died of the same disease.

During the course of their sessions, young Dora mentions to Freud that her father had a lover who Freud labels Frau K. and whose husband made sexual advances toward Dora, which she found repugnant, coming from the much older man. Her father seemed to ignore this in an attempt to preserve his own illicit relationship with Frau K., who, together with her husband, were friends of the family.

Because of this, Dora's father told her that the husband's advances were all a figment of her imagination. But later, Frau K.'s husband, Herr K., told a much different tale. Indeed, he had tried to seduce young Dora. Although Freud accepted Dora's account, his take on it was a series of specious leaps at best. Instead of accepting Dora's valid repugnance for a much older man, Freud insists that she was repressing both her own love for Herr K., as well as an incestuous love of her father, and at the same time a homosexual attraction for Frau K.

From a more medically based perspective, Dora's father had in fact developed tuberculosis when she was six years old, a disease he was never able to entirely shake and from which he had constant relapses punctuated by fever and coughing until his death in 1913. Tuberculosis characteristically doesn't do its greatest damage, for unknown reasons, between ages five and fifteen. Dora comes to Freud at age fourteen. Dora's mother also dies from tuberculosis. Freud doesn't chart this, feeling that it was insignificant. Dora begins to suffer her own lung involvement at age eight with constant episodes of shortness of breath that seem to assuage with enforced rest for a six-month period. Her family doctor, knowing full well the stigma of even mentioning the possibility of tuberculosis, puts down that the shortness of breath was from "nervous causes."[7]

At age twelve, Dora's shortness of breath is joined by spasmodic episodes of "nervous" coughing, generally lasting three to five weeks and associated with loss of voice. Rather than attribute Dora's coughing spells to TB or her voice loss to a tubercular attack on the sixth recurrent laryngeal nerve, Freud immediately seizes upon a series of hypotheses that few besides himself could even fathom, much less have thought up.

Dora's coughing, claims Freud, expressed her sexual longing for her father and her rivalry with Frau K. regarding this. And her throat irritation and consequent coughing was, Freud maintained, a combined symbolization of her desire to take Frau K.'s place in performing fellatio on her father. As if this wasn't enough, supposedly, the ceaseless coughing also expressed Dora's desire to replace her father in his affair with Frau K. Freud thereby assumes that Dora has lesbian tendencies as well. Later Dora married in what proved to be an entirely heterosexual relationship without a mention of any homoerotic tendencies whatsoever.

"In 1918, Sigmund Freud, during a speech at the Fifth International Congress of Psychoanalysis in Budapest, insisted that "The neuroses threaten public health no less than tuberculosis." But he never saw the possible interconnection between the two. Or if he did, he chose not to speak of it."

At the time of its release, *Studies on Hysteria* was not well received by European medicine. And it was not until years later that psychoanalysis was recognized as a legitimate psychiatric tool.

In 1918, Sigmund Freud, during a speech at the Fifth International Congress of Psychoanalysis in Budapest, insisted that "The neuroses threaten public health no less than tuberculosis."[8]

But he never saw the possible interconnection between the two. Or if he did, he chose not to speak of it.

43

1. Freud, S., and Freud, E. L. *Letters of Sigmund Freud.* New York. Courier Dover Publications, 1992, 68.
2. Freud, S. *Beyond the Pleasure Principle.* Trans by James Strachey. New York. Liveright Publishing Corporation. 1961
3. Cardanus, J. *Ii, de phthisis.* J. G. Schenck, Editor. Francofurti: Sumpt. J. Beyeri Publishers, 1665, 265.
4. Eysenck, H. J., Mead, M., and Eysenck, S.B.G. *Decline and Fall of the Freudian Empire.* Piscataway, New Jersey: Transaction Publishers, 2004.
5. Thornton, E. M. *Freud and Cocaine: The Freudian Fallacy.* London: Blond & Briggs, 1983.
6. Ellenberger, H. F. *The Discovery of the Unconscious: The History and Evolution of Dynamic Psychiatry.* New York: Basic Books, 1970.
7. Wenegrat, B. *Theater of Disorder: Patients, Doctors, and the Construction of Illness.* New York: Oxford University Press, 2001, 100.
8. Danto, E. A. *Freud's Free Clinics: Psychoanalysis and Social Justice 1918–38.* New York: Columbia University Press, 2005, 17.

10. CHILD PSYCHIATRY SERVICE, JOHNS HOPKINS UNIVERSITY HOSPITAL, PEDIATRIC DIVISION, BALTIMORE, 1934

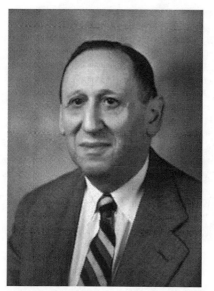

Figure 10. Dr. Leo Kanner (1955). Born June 13, 1894; Died April 3, 1981 (aged 86). By 1943 Kanner published a study of 11 children

identified with early infantile autism which became known as Kanner Syndrome. This seminal paper, entitled "Autistic Disturbances of Affective Contact", together with the work of Hans Asperger, formed the basis of the modern study of autism. However neither Kanner nor Asperger came down strongly in favor of an organic or infectious cause.

Kanner, with little use for medical diagnostics himself, seems made-to-order for Meyer. Kanner will laud Meyer for shifting the emphasis of psychiatry "from organs and their diseases to patients as improperly functioning persons."[1]

But diseased organs can themselves lead to improperly functioning persons.

Kanner never really seemed that interested in "organs and their diseases". While still in Berlin finishing his medical education, his lowest grade on his finals is as the result of being unable to diagnosis the then premier infectious brain disorder leading to mental symptoms. Neurologist Karl Bonhoeffer documents that Kanner misinterpreted the symptoms of *tabes dorsalis*, a neurologic end-stage syphilis of the brain and nervous system.[2]

Not really attracted to being a general internist, and still in Berlin, Kanner gravitates into the then new and relatively limited field of electrocardiography, or EKG tracings of the heart's rhythms.

"Kanner, with little use for medical diagnostics himself, seems made-

to-order for Meyer. Kanner will laud Meyer for shifting the emphasis of psychiatry "from organs and their diseases to patients as improperly functioning persons.""

Once at Johns Hopkins, Kanner writes his first edition of *Child Psychiatry* in 1935, borrowing the name from the German term *Kinderpsychiatrie*. And by 1943, bent upon making his mark, he discovers a "new" syndrome. Without mention of Bleuler, who originated the word *"autism"*, Kanner uses it to describe what he feels to be a novel psychiatric illness in children, emphasizing an "autistic aloneness" and "insistence on sameness." Ironically, Kanner, known to rant and rage over mere psychiatric labels without treatment, creates another one: autism.

1. Kanner, L. The Pediatric-Psychiatric Alliance. *Can Med Assoc Journal*, 38, no. 1 (January 1938): 71–74.
2. Neumarker, K. Leo Kanner: His Years in Berlin, 1906–24. The Roots of Autistic Disorder. in *History of Psychiatry*, 14, no. 54, part 2 (June 2003): 205–18.

11. OFFICE OF THE DIRECTOR, DEPARTMENT OF MEDICAL GENETICS, NEW YORK STATE PSYCHIATRIC INSTITUTE, JULY 1936

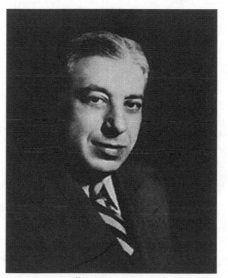

Figure 11. Dr. Franz J. Kallmann Born July 24, 1897 Neumarkt, Silesia - Died May 12, 1965 (aged 67), New York. Kallmann was

one of the first to study the genetic basis of psychiatric disorder. He spent most of his career in New York, where he pioneered the use of twin studies in the assessment of the relative roles of heredity and the environment in the pathogenesis of psychiatric disease.

Leo Kanner and Franz J. Kallmann had a couple of things in common. Both had connections with the University of Berlin. Kallmann worked for four years at Berlin's psychiatric institute under the same Karl Friedrich Bonhoeffer who graded a portion of Kanner's final exams. Although Kanner is only three years older than Kallmann, and Kanner is trained in internal medicine, both would move quickly upon their arrival to the United States to make their impact on psychiatry.

Landing in New York, Kallmann establishes the Medical Genetics Department of the New York State Psychiatric Institute. From then on, one thing is certain: With Franz J. Kallmann, American psychiatry got much more of the hereditary patterns in mental disease than it was willing to accept or pursue. Prominent British geneticist Penrose judged Kallmann's work unconvincing.

A year after Kanner writes *Child Psychiatry*, Kallmann becomes interested in twins and their genetic disposition. But there arises an inconvenient truth: Identical twins, who have virtually the same DNA, do not always develop the same mental disorders.

Kallmann focuses on what he calls the "genetics of schizophrenia." In a lecture, he finds it desirable to prevent the reproduction of relatives of patients with schizophrenia. He defines them as undesirable from a eugenic point of view, especially at the beginning of their reproductive years.

By 1938, Kallmann, who escaped Nazi Germany because he was half Jewish, has doubled down, calling for the "legal power" to sterilize "tainted children and siblings of schizophrenics" and to prevent marriages involving "schizoid eccentrics and borderline cases." In his mind, Kallmann feels the need to stamp out every recessive gene behind schizophrenia.[1] It was a thought that began incubating in him while he was still in Germany. Leo Kanner is appalled by Kallmann's thoughts and words. He sees dangerous implications. This time he is correct.

Kallmann is a zealot in every sense of the word. He finds a genetic basis for just about everything. He proclaims that human tuberculosis is genetically based. His agenda in doing so is quite transparent.

"In his mind, Kallmann feels the need to stamp out every recessive gene behind schizophrenia."

Proponents like Kallmann for a "genetic" or "hereditary" view of mental illness have always relied on identical twin studies. In these, if there is a heavy degree of "concordance" —meaning that if both identical twins come down with the illness—it is supposed that "genetic" influences are involved. This is so, especially if at the same time fraternal twins show a much lower rate in being "concordant for" — or contracting—the same disease.

But it was also known that an infectious disease like tuberculosis brought in the same numbers in identical twin studies as did schizophrenia or autism, putting the accuracy of such twin studies deeply in question.

In fact, it was Kallmann[2, 3] himself who found that approximately 85 percent of identical (homozygous) twins had the same disease (were concordant) if their co-twin had either tuberculosis or schizophrenia.

Kallmann's study for the hereditary basis of schizophrenia is published in 1938. It acknowledges his long-time boss and Nazi mentor Ernst Rudin.[4] While still in Germany, Kallmann saw Rudin catapulted to director of the Kaiser Wilhelm Institute for Psychiatry and its eugenics division through Rockefeller Foundation money, creating the medical specialty known as psychiatric genetics. Rudin was not only assisted by Kallmann but another protégé named Otmar

Verschuer. Back in Germany, Rudin, a year later, sees to it that the German version of Kallmann's book is used by the Nazi T4 Unit as a blueprint for the murder of mental patients and "defectives," many of them children. 250,000 are killed under this program, by gas and lethal injection. The Rockefeller-Rudin operation had become a section of the Nazi state. Rudin was now head of its Racial Hygiene Society.

Meanwhile, in the United States, geneticist Franz Kallmann becomes an early leader of the American Society of Human Genetics, a true pioneer in the study of the genetic basis of psychiatric disorders.

Kallmann's American Society of Human Genetics organizes the Human Genome Project—the most ambitious project ever dealing with basic genetics. In 1988, Congress provides funds for the National Institutes of Health and other groups to begin mapping out human DNA. The project began officially on October 1, 1990, with a projected budget of $3 billion over the next fifteen years.

As B. W. Richards points out, advances regarding the discovery of genetic markers for diseases such as autism, Down syndrome, and schizophrenia, although good for diagnostics, have done little to get at the actual cause of such chromosomal aberrations. Richards: "Despite dramatic advances in the fields of biochemistry and cytogenetics, revealing many new causes of mental retardation, a large proportion of mentally retarded patients are still undiagnosable in respect of etiology [cause]."[5]

What did result, thanks to such take-no-prisoners actions like Kallmann's, was that bacteriology was purposely confined to a specialty of medicine outside the schools of biology, botany, and zoology, in no small part responsible for bacteriology's slow acceptance.

Bacteriologists, in retaliation, steered clear and gave no credence to any of the proclamations of geneticists. Unbelievably, the situation had gotten so out of hand that, as late as 1945, bacteriologist Rene Dubos, discoverer of the first antibiotic ever, had to muster all of the courage in him to name his milestone paper "The Bacterial Cell." Such are and always have been the politics of medicine.

"As B. W. Richards points out, advances regarding the discovery of genetic markers for diseases such as autism, Down syndrome, and schizophrenia, although good for diagnostics, have done little to get at the actual cause of such chromosomal aberrations."

1. Muller-Hill, B. *Murderous Science: Elimination by Scientific Selection of Jews, Gypsies, and Others in Germany, 1933–1945.* Woodbury, NY: Cold Spring Harbor Laboratory Press, 1988, 11, 31, 42–43, 70.
2. Kallman, F. J., and Resiner, D. Twin Studies on the Significance of Genetic Factors in Tuberculosis. *Am. Rev. Tuberc., 47* (1943): 549.
3. Kallman, F. J. The Genetic Theory of Schizophrenia. Analysis of 691 Twin Index Families. *Am. J. Psychiat., 103* (1946): 309.
4. Torrey, E. F., and Yolken, R. H. Psychiatric Genocide: Nazi Attempts to Eradicate Schizophrenia. *Schizophr Bull.,* September 2009.
5. Richards, B. W. Recent Advances in Medical Knowledge of Causes of Mental Retardation. *Can Med Assoc J., 89,* no. 24 (December 14, 1963): 1230–33.

12. OFFICE OF THE DIRECTOR OF CHILD PSYCHIATRY, JOHNS HOPKINS HOSPITAL, BALTIMORE, 1943

To make certain that his theory sticks, Kanner cherry-picks eleven children, leaving out those presently with seizures or mental retardation even though these are very much in today's autistic spectrum. Some studies have mental retardation occurring in approximately two-thirds of individuals with autism and seizures in approximately one-third.

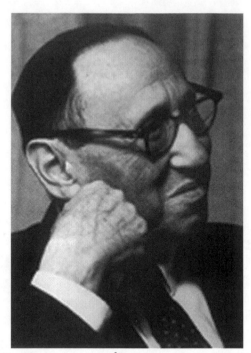

Figure 12. Dr. Leo Kanner. His first autistic case was Donald T. first
seen in October, 1938, at the age of 5 years. In August, 1937, Donald
was placed in a tuberculosis preventorium in order to provide
for him "a change of environment".

Kanner produces a thirty-three-page medically sketchy
paper.[1] He outlines eleven case histories, all the while convincing himself that, despite findings such as a history of
seizures, which could point to a brush with serious disease,
his subjects' problems were purely psychiatric or behavioral. At the same time, he says that, unlike childhood schizophrenia, autism is the result of "inborn autistic disturbances
of affective contact" —a kind of congenital lack of interest in
other people. Yet most of his children are thought to be deaf,

neither talking nor responding if questioned, and could have severe cranial nerve disruption from a previous or present serious central nervous system infection.

"Physically," Kanner insists, despite findings that suggest otherwise, "the children were essentially normal." But five out of his eleven subjects, through measurement "had relatively large heads," which could indicate possible degrees of hydrocephalous. Hydrocephalous, also known as "water on the brain," is a medical condition in which there is an abnormal accumulation of cerebrospinal fluid in the ventricles, or deep cavities, in the brain. This may cause increased intracranial pressure inside the skull and progressive enlargement of the head, seizures, and mental disability. Not uncommon, one of its causes in infants is perinatal infection affecting the brain and nervous system. At one time, the diagnosis of acute hydrocephalus was so commonly associated with tuberculous meningitis that the terms were used interchangeably.

"Kanner produces a thirty-three-page medically sketchy paper. He outlines eleven case histories, all the while convincing himself that, despite findings such as a history

of seizures, which could point to a brush with serious disease, his subjects' problems were purely psychiatric or behavioral."

But apparently of more concern to Kanner were the children's parents: "In the whole group, there are very few really warmhearted fathers or mothers." Kanner in general felt that disturbed children often were the product of parents who were highly organized, rational, and cold, "just happening to defrost enough to have a child."[2]

When, in his first case, Kanner finds out through Donald T.'s mother that the child had been placed in a "tuberculosis preventorium" for "a change of environment," Kanner never questions her as to why, but notes that while in the tuberculosis preventorium, he exhibited a "disinclination to play with children." Kanner will later relate that "the mother gave Donald little attention because "she feared he would give her tuberculosis" and casually dismisses this by adding, "which he did not have."[3] But in order to be sent to a preventorium, Donald T. must have had a positive TB skin test, which was not mentioned; nor was it mentioned what other tests were performed to rule out that the child did indeed not have tuberculosis.

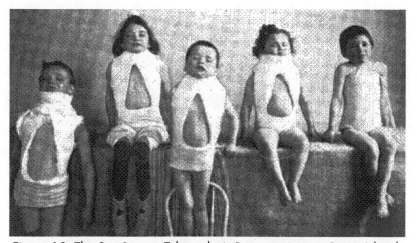

Figure 13. The Sea Breeze Tuberculosis Preventorium at Coney Island, Brooklyn, New York: where poor children who had been determined to have contracted tuberculosis in tenement city neighborhoods could go. Some of these children were fitted with casts there. Picture appeared in "The Seashore and Fresh Air Treatment at Sea Breeze Hospital", presented by John W. Brannan, M.D. at the *Sixth International Congress on Tuberculosis*, Vol. 2; W. F. Fell Company, 1908. American Preventoriums were designed to protect children from the ravages of TB and existed from 1909 to approximately 1970.

"The imprecise designation "pretubercular" was used to designate children with positive skin tests who didn't seem to have active disease. These were the children targeted for preventoriums."

All but forgotten, tuberculosis preventoriums were America's answer to preventing tuberculosis epidemics among the urban poor. This was accomplished by ripping "pretubercular" children from their homes and placing them into residential institutions.[4] From the beginning of the twentieth century and well into it, such primitive "preventoriums" were seen as the only solution to break the chain in a disease that, by 1900, had killed at least 15 percent of urban populations, with no treatment in sight. By 1907, von Pirquet came up with a children's tuberculin skin test with all the flaws of our present adult tuberculin skin test. Not only were false negative tests done on seriously infected children whose immune systems could simply not muster a positive skin reaction, but even when the test proved positive, it was often impossible to distinguish mere previous exposure from active disease. Nevertheless, the imprecise designation "pretubercular" was used to designate children with positive skin tests who didn't seem to have active disease. These were the children targeted for preventoriums.

Kanner knows from the onset that his definition of "autism" will be challenged, on many levels. Even among psychiatrists presented with these same children, responses would include mentally retarded or schizophrenic.

The fact was that, psychiatrically, all would be considered by many as having a form of childhood schizophrenia. To make the differentiation stick, Kanner emphasizes "extreme solitude from the very beginning of life" and a preserved intelligence. But many of the developmentally disabled children that Down had studied had normal intelligence also and certainly did not appear to have mental retardation.[5] Kanner argues that the children in his study, unlike schizophrenics, did not seem to have delusions or hallucinations. In addition, he says, schizophrenia doesn't emerge in as early as the thirty months after birth that autism seemed to.

But more tellingly, in 1949, Kanner vacillates, admitting that he sees no need for his "infantile autism" to be separated from schizophrenia.[6] The American Psychiatric Association (APA) balks in accommodation and decades later still won't acknowledge autism as anything other than just that: "schizophrenia, childhood type."[7] By then, Kanner deplores the APA's decision.[8] Yet despite this, until 1980, Kanner's autism is not autism; it is childhood schizophrenia.[9]

"But more tellingly, in 1949, Kanner vacillates, admitting that he sees no need for his "infantile autism" to be separated from schizophrenia."

One year after the APA's 1968 decision, prominent Bellevue child psychiatrist Lauretta Bender argues that children with autism generally grow up to have schizophrenia anyway. And on top of that, despite the ever-increasing rallying cry by American psychiatric gurus as to childhood schizophrenia's extreme rarity, Bender documents thousands of cases of it while at Bellevue.[10] German psychiatry, which long maintained its influence over Europe, and the Soviet and Eastern Bloc countries also insisted that childhood autism is the initial form of schizophrenia, with development into schizophrenia more or less inevitable.

Moreover, some in the field understood that clear and unmistakable evidence of the autistic disorder could be found in J. Langdon Down's 1887 "developmental" form of mental retardation, which Down attributed mostly to tuberculosis in the child's parents.[11, 12] The stage was set for a battle royal.

1. Kanner, L. Problems of Nosology and Psychodynamics of Early Infantile Autism. *American Journal of Orthopsychiatry*, 19 (1949): 416–26.
2. Kanner, L. Medicine: The Child Is Father. *Time*, July 25, 1960.
3. Kanner, L., Rodriguez A., and Ashenden, B. How Far Can Autistic Children Go in Matters of Social Adaptation?

Journal of Autism and Childhood Schizophrenia, 2, no. 1 (1972): 9–33.

4. Connolly, C. A. *Saving Sickly Children: The Tuberculosis Preventorium in American Life, 1909–1970*. New Brunswick, NJ: Rutgers University Press, 2008.

5. Treffert, D. A. Dr. Down and 'Developmental Disorders' *J. Autism Dev Disorder*, 36, no. 7 (October 2006): 965–66.

6. Kanner, L. Problems of Nosology and Psychodynamics of Early Infantile Autism *American Journal of Orthopsychiatry* 19, (1949):416-26.

7. American Psychiatric Association. *Diagnostic and Statistical Manual of Mental Disorders*, 2nd ed. Washington, DC: American Psychiatric Association, 1968.

8. Neumarker, K. Leo Kanner: His Years in Berlin, 1906–24. The Roots of Autistic Disorder. *History of Psychiatry*, 14, no. 54, part 2 (June 2003): 205–18.

9. American Psychiatric Association. *Diagnostic and Statistical Manual of Mental Disorders*, 3rd ed. Washington, DC: American Psychiatric Association, 1980.

10. Bender, L. A Longitudinal Study of Schizophrenic Children with Autism. *Hospital and Community Psychiatry*, 20, no. 8 (1969): 230–37.

11. Down, J.L.H. Observations on an Ethnic Classification of Idiots. *London Hosp Clin Lects Reps*, 3 (1806): 259–62.

12. Down, J. L. *On Some of the Mental Affections of Childhood and Youth*. London: J & A Churchill, 1887.

13. JOHNS HOPKINS DEPARTMENT OF PATHOLOGY, BALTIMORE, 1946

Though his office was but a short distance away from Leo Kanner's, Johns Hopkins TB pathologist Arnold Rich lived in a completely different world. In Rich's world, there were no psychiatric hypotheticals, no diagnoses not verifiable by laboratory reagents and microscopic findings.

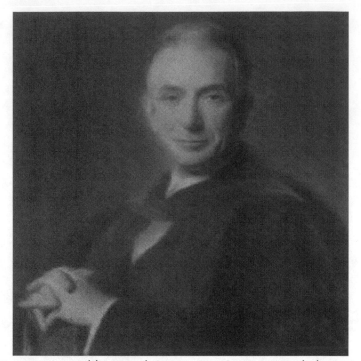

Figure 14. Arnold Rice Rich [1893-1968]. Became Pathologist-in-Chief of the Johns Hopkins Hospital after William Henry Welch. His continued research clarified the pathogenesis of the spread of the tubercle bacilli in the body and revolutionized the concept of the disease "tuberculosis" and its myriad manifestations, culminating in his *The Pathogenesis of Tuberculosis,* in 1944, revised in 1951 and subsequently translated into Spanish and Japanese.

Although it appeared that Rich and Kanner worked in completely different arenas, at times they unknowingly touched directly on one another's work, but never more closely than when Rich began to focus on perinatal infectious disease.

Rich was a teaching dynamo at Johns Hopkins, completing his authoritative *Pathogenesis of Tuberculosis* in 1944,[1] with a second edition in 1951. It took him nine years to compile and still remains a model of what a scientific monograph should be.

By virtue of his astute powers of observation, Rich had always stood out from the rest, even at Johns Hopkins. His name remains on the lung condition called Hamman-Rich syndrome, and the small tuberculous masses (tuberculomas) that metastasized, not infrequently, to, among other areas, the human brain, and became immortalized as "Rich's foci". He was also the first to describe the high prevalence of occult prostate cancer in elderly men as well as the first to describe widespread vascular obstruction in the lungs in children with the hereditary heart condition called Tetralogy of Fallot.

During Rich's tenure, much as in the past, the prevailing emphasis at Johns Hopkins laboratory research was either with the living or recently deceased, but the way in which Phipps psychiatry under Meyer neglected its bench work research gave it a somewhat remote character to the rest of Johns Hopkins, preventing closer association.

In addition, it seemed that Meyer's protégé, Leo Kanner was looking only at the very tip of the same iceberg that John Langdon Down had come to grips with so long ago. When Kanner spoke of an "inborn" condition affecting mentation, Rich, as well as Down previously, had a fairly good idea of what he was speaking about, and to Rich it was no more a condition caused by heredity than the nonsensical documents that crossed his desk weekly claiming human TB to be hereditary or caused by the wrong genes.

Rich, like Down, knew that TB was the most common cause of death from a single infectious agent in young children and neonates,[2] commonly attacking their central nervous system.[3] The Germans had their own name for childhood tuberculosis, *kindertuberkulose*, and in the many children who survived, besides leaving their tiny bodies gnarled, nearly 20 to 25 percent manifested mental retardation and psychiatric disorders.[4] And for various reasons, many did survive – leaving in its wake, among other conditions- Down syndrome, the autistic and the 'mentally disabled'.

"A neurologist friend had confided in Rich that Kanner's autism seemed more like a disease caused by postencephalitic phenomena than anything else."

So until this significant pool of infected neonates, infants, and toddlers was fully evaluated for such protean mental complications, Arnold Rich truly couldn't understand psychiatrist's fussing over "inborn" features of a "psychiatric" disease, whether labeled autism or anything else that very possibly was caused by organic infection. It just didn't make sense.

A neurologist friend had confided in Rich that Kanner's autism seemed more like a disease caused by postencephalitic phenomena than anything else. Rich knew that tuberculosis was fully capable of causing such an encephalitis, described by one pediatric infectious disease specialist as being indolent or slow to develop and heal, often as painlessly as any other central nervous infection around.[5]

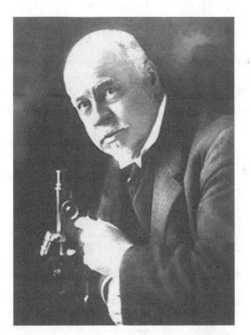

Figure 15. William Henry Welch [1850-1934] The first dean of the Johns Hopkins University School of Medicine. Often referred to as "the Dean of American Medicine". He was convinced that the maternal to fetal transmission of tuberculosis was common.

71

Rich looked up at the picture of William Henry Welch (1850–1934). Welch had been both Rich's predecessor at Hopkins Department of Pathology, as well as dean of medicine and founder of the Johns Hopkins University Medical School. Welch was unique. Welch was different. He was a mover and a shaker, an organizational genius who would single-handedly force US medicine up to and eventually beyond what they had in Europe. A bacteriologist and a pathologist, Welch would one day be called the dean of American medicine. During his watch American life expectancy would jump by at least twenty years. And William Henry Welch would be a major factor in that leap.

Rich was proud both of the association and to have personally known the physician considered both the father of American medicine and one of its most influential members. Welch had studied in Germany under the great masters, including stints with Koch, Cohnheim, and psychiatrist and neurologist Meynert. Welch therefore well realized the importance of seeking out diseased tissue in the mentally ill. Meynert decried those like Kraepelin and Meyer, who seemed preoccupied with labeling symptoms instead of going after the real tissue cause of brain or central nervous system illness.[6] And having also worked with Koch, Welch held a keen appreciation for the destruction, both inside and outside of the mind, that tuberculosis could cause.

With regard to the immediate problem in front of him, Rich had read Knoph's review in which he said of Welch that "He too was of the opinion that a direct bacillary transmission, that is to say, prenatal infection [with tuberculosis], takes place much more frequently than believed." [7]

Like Rich, Knoph also knew that few fetal autopsies and exhaustive studies were done to prove fatal tuberculosis on dead fetuses. And those studies had to contend with the fact that tuberculosis, a microbe that grew only with sufficient oxygen, was most often impossible to isolate in the low-oxygen content of fetal blood or tissue. It's not that TB had any trouble surviving under low-oxygen conditions; it just did so in undetectable dormant forms, causing a diagnostic nightmare.

"With regard to the immediate problem in front of him, Rich had read Knoph's review in which he said of Welch that "He too was of the opinion that a direct bacillary transmission, that is to say, prenatal infection [with tuberculosis], takes place much more frequently than believed."

Rich questioned the wisdom of Welch in choosing someone like Adolph Meyer to run Hopkins's psychiatry. Meyer
seemed such a far cry from Johns Hopkins neurologist D.J.
McCarthy, previously on staff at Phipps Tuberculosis[8] and
an authority on tuberculosis of the nervous system in infants
and children. McCarthy knew not only that cerebral tuberculosis occurred with much greater frequency in infancy
and childhood than most realized, but reported a distinct
and causative relationship between tuberculosis and adoles-
cent schizophrenia itself. In fact, McCarthy's investigation at
Johns Hopkins Phipps Tuberculous Pavilion for the mentally
ill revealed that practically all of the patients isolated there
had schizophrenia. This seemed particularly relevant when
taken in light of Lauretta Bender's argument that children
with autism generally grow up to have schizophrenia anyway.[9] McCarthy was far from the first investigator to link
schizophrenia with TB.

Although eventually the term *childhood schizophrenia*
was displaced altogether regarding autism, there remained
those children who displayed both the early-appearing
social and communicative deficits characteristic of autism
and the emotional instability and disordered thought processes that resembled schizophrenia.

Rich wondered if either Kanner or Meyer had as extensive a knowledge of the infectious orientation of German

psychiatry as did pathologist William Henry Welch, who once walked with its giants.

1. Rich, A. R. *The Pathogenesis of Tuberculosis.* Springfield, IL: Charles C. Thomas, 1946.
2. Walia, R., and Hoskyns, W. Tuberculous Meningitis in Children: Problem to Be Addressed Effectively with Thorough Contact Tracing. *Eur J Pediatr.*, 159, no. 7 (July 2000): 535–38.
3. Weaker, N. J. Jr., and Connor, J. D. Central Nervous System Tuberculosis in Children: A Review of 30 Cases. *Pediatr Infect Dis J,* 9 (1990): 539–43.
4. Garg, P. K. Tuberculosis of the Central Nervous System. *Post grad Med J, 75* (1999): 133–40.
5. Gutierrez, K. M., and Prober, C. G. Encephalitis Postgraduate Medicine, 103, no. 3 (March 1998): 123–25, 129–30, 140–43.
6. Meynert, T. Uber die Nothwendigkeit und Tragweitge einer anatomischen Richtung in der Psychiatrie. *Wiener Medizinische Wochenschrift,* 18 (May 1968): 573–76.
7. Knoph, Adolphus. The Period of Life at Which Infection from Tuberculosis Occurs Most Frequently. *American Journal of Public Health,* 6, no. 9 (September 1915): 934–52.
8. McCarthy, D. J. Tuberculous Affectations of the Nervous System in Infancy and Childhood. In *Tuberculosis in*

Infancy and Childhood, edited by T. N. Kelynack, 43–54. New York: William Wood Publishers, 1908.

9. Bender, L. A Longitudinal Study of Schizophrenic Children with Autism. *Hospital and Community Psychiatry,* 20, no. 8 (1969): 230–37.

14. PSYCHIATRIC ASYLUMS ON THE EUROPEAN AND AMERICAN CONTINENTS, LATE NINETEENTH CENTURY

When Johns Hopkins pathologist William Henry Welch studied under psychiatrist Meynert, it was in the late nineteenth century, a time of fear that tuberculosis would destroy the entire civilization of Europe. It was also when the first massive increase in psychiatric illness and confinement to mental asylums occurred.[1]

And although there was a sociological shift of patients going from family care and poorhouses to asylums, this in itself could not account for the inexorable increase in asylum census. To distinguished psychiatrist and writer E. Fuller

Torrey, severe psychiatric illnesses such as schizophrenia were comparatively new diseases, less than 250 years old, the confinement for which, even as a college student, reminded Torrey of the tuberculosis sanitariums of a slightly earlier era.[2]

During this time frame, there was no autism as understood by Kanner, just the autism Bleuler used to describe schizophrenia. Nor was there the capacity to do a proof-of-concept biostatistical analysis showing significant genetic overlap in humans with autism, schizophrenia and tuberculosis. Rather autism and schizophrenia were simply considered as one with infectious concepts brought forward still being revisited by various authors today. [3,4]

In nineteenth-century asylums, the upward spiral became obvious. By 1884, in Germany, Karl Kahlbaum, perhaps the most underrated psychiatrist in history and the true originator of US outcome-based psychiatric classification, first described schizophrenia as a separate entity. Kahlbaum: "It must be the experience of all psychiatric institutions that the number of youthful patients has recently undergone a considerable increase."[5] It was between 1700 and 1900, that tuberculosis was responsible for the deaths of approximately one billion (one thousand million) human beings. The annual death rate from TB when Koch discovered its cause was an incredible seven million people per year.

"Almost unheard of in the medical literature before this, chronic delusions and hallucinations— such as hearing voices—became common in asylum admissions at the same time Clouston, by 1892, was documenting them in mental illness as a result of a killer pandemic of tuberculosis."

There were others who also saw this nineteenth-century groundswell of mental illness as representing something new, including auditory hallucinations, as never witnessed before. Historians like Hare and Wilkins, among others, point out that it was only then that schizophrenia, with its hallucinations and delusions, was really even mentioned, representing no small part of the late-nineteenth-century psychiatric flare ups.[6,7]

Almost unheard of in the medical literature before this, chronic delusions and hallucinations—such as hearing voices—became common in asylum admissions at the same time Clouston, by 1892, was documenting them in mental illness as a result of a killer pandemic of tuberculosis.[8]

Max Jacobi, the originator of the school of thought that held that infectious illness led to mental illness, was the first to ascribe characteristic symptoms for this associated with tuberculosis.[9] Just as autism was thought to be a disease of "affect" or emotion by Kanner, Jacobi in particular considered an unpredictable, emotional (affective) changeability as characteristic of, and at times even diagnostic for, latent, undiagnosed TB.

Incredibly, Greding found pulmonary tuberculosis during autopsy in 70 percent of mental defectives and in 50 percent of the mentally affected with seizure disorders.[10] Seizures, not uncommon in autism, occur in 20 to 30 percent of its patients based on the majority of studies.[11]

"Just as autism was thought to be a disease of "affect" or emotion by Kanner, Jacobi in particular considered an unpredictable, emotional (affective) changeability as characteristic of, and at times even diagnostic for, latent, undiagnosed TB."

Barr spoke about the relationship between tuberculosis and mental defectiveness at the Sixth International Tuberculosis Congress held in Washington, DC, in 1908.[12] There, Jacques Moreau expressed his belief that epilepsy and the convulsive disorders were derived from tuberculosis. A year previously, Anglade spoke not only on how tuberculosis caused epilepsy in infants and the young, but how such epileptics eventually became mentally defective through sclerotic brain changes caused by the disease.[13]

Subsequently, Baruk discovered that when either proteins extracted from tuberculosis or the spinal fluid taken from people with schizophrenia were introduced into healthy animals, a condition called catalepsy occurred, in which the body and its functions seemed frozen in time. Catalepsy is associated not only with one form of schizophrenia but with epilepsy itself.[14] Patients with catatonia, an extreme form of withdrawal in which the individual retreats into a completely immobile state, can also exhibit catalepsy. Wing related in 2000 that the incidence of catatonia could be as high as 17 percent in adolescents with autism.[15]

Historically prominent Viennese pathologist Ernst Löwenstein decided to take things a step beyond. Having developed a potato flour-and egg-based tuberculosis growth media, still in use today, he set about to prove that TB could be cultured from the blood of patients with schizophrenia.[16]

Yet despite nine independent confirmative studies finding either the tuberculosis bacillus itself or it's much harder to stain yet more common viral forms, other studies couldn't confirm these results. Whether this was from defective laboratory procedure or from the difficulty in staining and culturing viral (or cell-wall-deficient forms) of tuberculosis remains, to this day, unknown. What is known is that unde-terred and in answer to these negative studies, Weeber,[17] Melgar,[18] and Löwenstein[19] again found tuberculosis in the blood of schizophrenic patients—findings which, to this day, remain unaddressed.

As far back as 1769, Scotsman Robert Whytt, reporting on approximately twenty cases, described the localization of tuberculosis in the meninges, membranes that cover the brain and spinal cord.[20] Realizing that the localization of tuberculosis there was often associated with mental distur-bances, Whytt gave us the first description of tuberculous meningitis, at that time called *morbus cerebralis Whyttii*. In describing the disease, Whytt noticed not only small masses called "tubercles" in the brain tissue but hydrocephalus, an excess of "water in the brain."

A duct system circulates fluid in the brain and spinal cord. The meninges that cover the brain manufacture and con-tain a cerebrospinal fluid that circulates through channels of deep cisterns in the brain and then down the spinal cord and back to the brain. A block in this circulation, whether from a congenital condition or disease, can lead to an increase of cerebrospinal fluid around the brain. In infants and young children, because the bones of their skulls are still unfused, this can result in an enlargement of the head. No matter the age, mental disturbances and even retardation can result as complications of such hydrocephalus. So intertwined was hydrocephalus with tuberculosis that medical experts by the end of the nineteenth century considered acute hydrocephalus as just another name for tuberculous meningitis.[21] Since 1854, Wunderlich recognized that psychotic episodes, including schizophrenia, could be caused by small masses of tuberculosis (tubercles) in the brain.[22] But only as time passed, did it became more obvious just how commonly this occurs. The tubercles of tuberculosis, which often form masses called tuberculomas, are launched through the bloodstream to the brain and are often found in infants and adults with no neurologic symptoms. But Marie documented symptomatic cases of tubercles as a cause of psychosis such as schizophrenia.[23] TB meningitis was just the tip of the iceberg, and other investigators, as early as 1908, uncovered a more generalized inflammation of the brain matter, tuberculous encephalitis, "as also being behind specific psychosis.[24] So the term *tuberculous meningoencephalitis* was considered more accurate than just *tuberculous meningitis*.

"TB meningitis was just the tip of the iceberg, and other investigators, as early as 1908, uncovered a more generalized inflammation of the brain matter, tuberculous encephalitis, "as also being behind specific psychosis. So the term tuberculous meningoencephalitis was considered more accurate than just tuberculous meningitis."

1. Torrey, E. F. Severe Psychiatric Disorders May Be Increasing. *Psychiatric Times*, 19, no. 4 (April 2002):2-4.
2. Torrey, E. F., and Miller, J. *The Invisible Plague: The Rise of Mental Illness from 1750 to the Present*. Piscataway, NJ: Rutgers University Press, 2002.
3. Ploeger, A., and Raijmakers, M. E. The Association between Autism and Errors in Early Embryogenesis: What Is the Causal Mechanism?. *Biol Psychiatry*, 67, no. 7 (April 2010): 602–7.
4. Rzhetsky, A., Wajngurt, D., Park, N., and Zheng, T. Probing Genetic Overlap among Complex Human Phenotypes. *Proceedings of the National Academy*

of *Sciences, Chicago,* 104, no. 28 (July 10, 2007): 11694–99.

5. Kessler, R. C., and McGonagle, K. A. Lifetime and 12-Month Prevalence of DSM-III-R Psychiatric Disorders in the United States. Results from the National Comorbidity Survey. *Arch Gen Psychiatry,* 51, no. 1 (January 1994: 8–19.

6. Hare, E. Was Insanity on the Increase? *BMJ,* 142 (1983): 439–45.

7. Wilkins, R. Hallucinations in Children and Teenagers Admitted to Bethlem Royal Hospital in the Nineteenth Century and Their Possible Relevance to the Incidence of Schizophrenia *Journal of Child Psychology and Psychiatry,* 28 (1987): 569–80.

8. Clouston, T. S. Phthisical Insanity *History of Psychiatry,* 64, no. 4 (December 2005: 479–95.

9. Jacobi, M. *Annalen der Irrenheilanstalt zu Siegburg.* Köln: Dumont & Schauberg, 1837.

10. Greding, J. *Sämmtliche medicinische Schriften,* Vol. 1, 277–350; Vol. 2, 145–62, 327–33. Greiz, Germany. C. W. Henning Publishers. Greiz: Henning, 1790-1.

11. Kagan-Kushnir, T., Roberts, W., and Snead, C. Screening Electroencephalograms in Autism Spectrum Disorders: Evidence-Based Guideline. *J Child Neurol,* 20, no. 3 (March 2005): 197–206.

12. Barr, M. W. The Relationship between Tuberculosis and Mental Defect. *Sixth International Congr. Tuberc. Washington, DC, 1908.* Philadelphia: Fell, 1908.

13. Anglade and Jacquin. Hérédo-tuberculose et idioties congénitales. *Encéphale,* 1 (1907): 136–57.

14. Baruk, H. *Psychiatric.* Paris: Masson, 1938.

15. Wing, L., and Shah, A. Catatonia in Autistic Spectrum Disorders. *Br. J. Psychiatry,* 176 (2000): 357–62.

16. Löwenstein, E. Das Vorkommen der Tuberkelbazillämie bei verschiedenen Krankheiten. *Münch. Med. Wschr.,* 78 (1931): 261–63.

17. Weeber, R. Ueber Blut- und Liquorbazillose. *Wien. Med Wschr.,* 87 (1937): 285–86.

18. Melger, R. Tuberculosis y psicosis. *Rev. Asoc. Méd. Argent.,* 57 (1943): 1061–64.

19. Löwenstein, E. Tubercle Bacilli in Spinal Fluid. *J. Nerv. Ment. Dis.,* 101 (1945): 576–82.

20. Whytt, R. *Observation on the Dropsy of the Brain.* Edinburgh, 1768.

21. *Encyclopedia Britannica.* Edited by H. Chisholm London: Cambridge University Press, 1911.

22. Wunderlich, C. A. *Handbuch der Pathologie und Therapie.* Stuttgart, Germany: Ebner & Seubert, 1854.

23. Marie, A. Tuberculose et psychose. *Bull. Soc. Méd. Paris,* 2 (1930): 457–61.

24. Lépine, J. Tuberculose-Encephalite. Psychoses. In *Sixth International Cong. Tuberc.,* Vol. 1, part 2. *Washington DC, 1908.* Philadelphia: Fell, 1908.

15. DEPARTMENT OF PATHOLOGY JOHNS HOPKINS, 1948

Arnold Rich was working on a problem that might have major implications toward Kanner's child psychiatry, but he was having a problem with regard to the frequency of maternal-to-fetal transfer of tuberculosis.[1] It was also an issue with seminal significance in addressing Down's developmental disorders, of which autism was a division. In fact, it was a topic that had been addressed by some of the greatest minds in medicine.

On the one hand, Rich knew that "It is now well established that tuberculous infection can be transmitted from mother to fetus through the placenta." He references Warthin, who in an article in the *Journal of Infectious Diseases*,[2] said it was common, and Siegel's study in the *American Review of Tuberculosis*.[3] Siegel documented infants that had died from the disease, one or two days after birth. Husted's study even included tubercular stillbirth.[4]

But to further establish the importance of a link between maternal and perinatal tuberculosis, Arnold Rich felt the need to go into the numbers involved in the general population. Of all the infectious diseases, TB was and always had been a disease of alarmingly large numbers.

Ever since Norris's original review, it had been known that, for some reason, pregnancy, especially late pregnancy, and child bearing itself dangerously reanimated any form of tuberculosis in a woman's body, no matter how silent.[5] Even latent TB with no symptoms, Norris mentions, could reactivate, percolating TB bacilli into the maternal bloodstream for transfer into the fetus. Thus, in the first half of the twentieth century, the method of choice for an expectant mother with proven TB was early termination of pregnancy.[6] Menstruation itself had a similar deleterious effect, causing its own flare up of tuberculosis in the body.

The numbers in front of Rich were incredible.

In a disease that, according to the World Health Organization, consistently kills more women of childbearing age than any other, the age at which female tuberculosis mortality began to rise above male mortality coincided with the average age of the onset of menstruation. But the age at which the rate of tuberculosis mortality really surpassed that of males coincided with the period during which over two-thirds of all pregnancies occurred.

Rich conservatively estimated that a little over two million women between the ages of eighteen and thirty were pregnant in 1940. And since the total US population for women of this age was approximately 17.7 million, it followed that one out of every eight women in the United States was pregnant in this age range, and one in ten bore living children. This not only produced a pool of 200,000 opportunities to reanimate dormant and often undiagnosed maternal tuberculosis, with its drastically increased female mortality rate, but, with such reactivation, the possibility for the transmission of that disease to the fetus and newborn.

"Ever since Norris's original review, it had been known that, for some reason, pregnancy, especially late pregnancy, and child bearing itself dangerously reanimated any form of tuberculosis in a woman's body, no matter how silent. Even latent

TB with no symptoms, Norris mentions, could reactivate, percolating TB bacilli into the maternal bloodstream for transfer into the fetus. Thus, in the first half of the twentieth century, the method of choice for an expectant mother with proven TB was early termination of pregnancy."

In such a reanimation of latent tuberculosis, it was also striking that TB meningitis—which is infrequent in adults but frequent in infants and toddlers—seemed to also noticeably increase in childbearing women from the reactivation of old deposits of cerebral tuberculosis.[7]

Rich already realized that, regarding TB's fatality in neonates, infants, and young children, there was a definite pattern. Tuberculosis was most fatal during the first year or two of life. After the second year, the death rate for infected toddlers fell markedly, probably through a greater ability to form protective antibodies between the ages of two and five than during infancy.[8] Though the disease was still deadly for the remainder of the first five years, by far the safest period was between five years and puberty, when the death rate from TB plummeted. Often termed the "golden age of resistance," for some reason, children between ages five and fifteen are more resistant to TB than adults and infants. It was an interesting fact, creating a possible theoretical underpinning for Bender's assertion as to how autistic involvement in the very young, hardest hit in the first thirty months, could come back as a related schizophrenia during adolescence, toward the end of the period of remarkable resistance to the disease.

It was thought at one time that newborns were completely devoid of resistance to tuberculosis.[9] But sufficient studies had since contradicted this notion. In Brailey's study at Rich's own Johns Hopkins Hospital, of sixty-five infants who became tuberculin positive during the first year of life, two-thirds were alive and well at the end of five years.[10] So the acquisition of tuberculosis by infants was not necessarily a death sentence. However, its complications, including those involving the brain and nervous system, could soon impact the individual for the rest of his or her life.

As to whether a not-uncommon tuberculous focus in the brain killed, Rich would soon find, was a matter of what he could only refer accurately to as what card players know as ' the luck of the draw'.

"As to whether a not-uncommon tuberculous focus in the brain killed, Rich would soon find, was a matter of what he could only refer accurately to as what card players know as 'the luck of the draw'."

It is not generally appreciated that the development of small, rounded nodules caused by tuberculosis, sometimes cheesy or "caseous" in the brain, is a relatively common occurrence in children and childhood tuberculosis. It is usually symptomless. Such small nodules often become arrested and encapsulated by the body's immune system. They are, to this day, called Rich's foci. Many of us unknowingly have them. But, stressed Rich, it is when small tubercle nodules happen to land in that part of the surface of the cerebral cortex near the meninges (covering of the brain), no matter how small, that serious troubles began. Such infectious nodules often extended into this protective covering through which cerebrospinal fluid percolates on its journey through the brain and into the spine. Such a discharge of tuberculosis into the spinal fluid of the meninges (in its subarachnoid space) can (and often does) lead to potentially fatal meningitis. The disease festers and spreads throughout the central nervous system. There need not be extensive infection, just one tiny nodule in the wrong place, near the meninges. On the other hand, the development of small tubercles deeper in the brain substance, though relatively common, often gave rise to no symptoms whatsoever. Rich himself had seen one-inch tuberculous masses lodged in a silent area of the brain that were seemingly entirely harmless.

A severe hypersensitivity reaction to just the tuberculo-protein thrown off in even a dormant tubercular infection could also occur in any tissue in the body, including the brain, in infants already hypersensitized to tuberculous pro-tein while in their mother's womb. Burn and Finley showed damage and death of cells as well as acute inflammation in the meninges in such instances.[11] The inflammation that resulted required no TB bacilli, just the sustained diffusion of the protein of the tuberculosis bacilli or its active split prod-ucts through the placenta into a previously sensitized infant.

Through it all, one thing was certain: Tuberculosis did not always kill. That infants could survive even a massive dose of tuberculosis was amply demonstrated in the tragedy called the Lubeck episode.[12] In the German city of Lübeck, of 251 infants mistakenly injected with large numbers of virulent human tubercular bacilli, incorrectly thought to be the TB vaccination called BCG, 71.3 percent survived.

"That infants could survive even a massive dose of tuberculosis was amply demonstrated in the tragedy called the Lübeck episode."

But the number of possible complications in those infants and children who survived TB's onslaught, including those to the brain and nervous system, Rich knew, would be enough to keep symptom-based psychiatry perturbed and under siege for some time to come.

1. Rich, A. R. *The Pathogenesis of Tuberculosis.* Springfield, IL: Chas C. Thomas, 1946.
2. Warthin, A. S., and Cowie, D.M. A Contribution in the Casuistry of Placental and Congenital Tuberculosis. *Journal of Infectious Diseases* 1 (1904): 140-169.
3. Siegel, M. Pathological Findings and Pathogenesis of Congenital Tuberculosis *American Review of Tuberculosis,* 29 (1934): 297-309.
4. Husted, E. Un cas de tuberculose millaire congenital. *Acta Path et Microbiol Scand,* Supp. 16 (1933): 163-171.
5. Norris, C. C. *Gynecological and Obstetrical Tuberculosis.* New York: D. Appleton, 1921.

6. Kobrinsky, S. Pregnancy and Tuberculosis. *Canad. M.A.J.*, 59 (November 1948): 462–64.

7. Whitney, J. S. *Facts and Figures about Tuberculosis.* [New York]: National Tuberculosis Association, 1931.

8. Halber, W., and Hirszfeld, H., and Mayzner, M. Beiträge zur Konstitutionsserologie; Untersuchungen über die Antikör perentstehung bei Kindern im Zusammenhang mit dem Alter. *Zschr. Immunforsch.*, 53 (1927): 391-418.

9. Cummins, S. L. Tuberculosis in Primitive Tribes and Its Bearing On the Tuberculosis of Civilized Communities. *International Journal of Public Health*, 1 (1920): 137.

10. Brailey, M. Mortality in Tuberculin Positive Infants. *Bull. Johns Hopkins Hosp.*, 59 (1936): 1-10.

11. Burn, C. G., and Finley, K. H. The Role of Hypersensitivity in the Production of Experimental Meningitis. *Journ. Exp. Med.*, 56 (1932): 203-21.

12. Moegling A. Die epidemiologie der Lubecker *sauglingstuberkulose. Arb Reichsges Amt,* 69, (1935):1-24.

16. UNIVERSITY OF PENNSYLVANIA DEPARTMENT OF PSYCHOLOGY, 1949

But psychiatry was already under siege. In 1949, psychologist Philip Ash, in a University of Pennsylvania postdoctoral dissertation, proved that three psychiatrists faced with a single patient and given identical information at the same moment in time were able to reach the same diagnostic conclusion only about 20 percent of the time.[1] Subsequently, Aaron T. Beck, one of the founders of cognitive-behavioral therapy, published a similar study in 1962 which, although it found psychiatric agreement a bit higher, at between 32 percent and 42 percent, still left doubts regarding the reliability of a psychiatric diagnosis in general.[2]

Added to this came the Rosenhan experiment, a well-known probe into the validity of psychiatric diagnosis conducted by Stanford University psychologist David Rosenhan in 1972.[3] Published in *Science* and entitled "On Being Sane in Insane Places," Rosenhan's study consisted of two parts. The first involved the use of mentally healthy associates or fake patients, who briefly pretended auditory hallucinations in an attempt to gain admission to twelve different psychiatric hospitals in five different US states. All of these mentally healthy persons were admitted and diagnosed with psychiatric disorders. All were also forced to admit they had mental illness and to take antipsychotic drugs as a condition for their release.

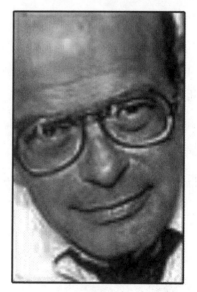

Dr. David L. Rosenhan [1929 – February 6, 2012] was an American psychologist best known for the Rosenhan experiment, a study challenging the validity of psychiatric diagnosis.

The second part of Rosenhan's experiment involved asking staff at a psychiatric hospital to detect fake patients in a group of people who were all mentally ill. No fake patients were sent to various psychiatric institutions in this phase of the Rosenhan experiment, yet staffs at these institutions falsely identified large numbers of actual mental patients as pretenders.

The study was considered an important and influential criticism of psychiatric diagnosis. Rosenhan concluded, "It is clear that we cannot distinguish the sane from the insane in psychiatric hospitals." The study also illustrated the dangers of depersonalization and the mere slapping on of a label that goes on in these institutions.

"Paul McHugh, former chair of psychiatry at Johns Hopkins, noticed that the DSM has "permitted groups of "experts" with a bias to propose the existence of conditions without anything more than a definition and a checklist of symptoms. "This is just how witches used to be identified.", he noted."

As a result of such intrusions, the American Psychiatric Association (APA) in 1973 asked psychiatrist Robert Spitzer to chair a classification task force to establish more precise medically oriented parameters. The problem was that such a classification would still be symptom or syndrome focused. The end result was a classification manual, along the lines of Emil Kraepelin's rejuvenated categorizing, entitled the *Diagnostic and Statistical Manual of Mental Disorders* (DSM), Third Edition, or *DSM-III*.[4] Though *DSM-III* was indeed more reliable than its predecessors, it still offered no clear definition of the *cause* of the many different "mental illnesses" it defined.[5] Without causes, the mere categorizing of psychiatric diseases did not mean that they were valid to begin with and not the result of direct physical illness. While the APA admitted it had no idea of what caused its manual's supposed "mental" illnesses; at the same time, it felt completely confident in its ability to diagnose and "treat" them.

Paul McHugh, former chair of psychiatry at Johns Hopkins, noticed that the *DSM* has "permitted groups of "experts" with a bias to propose the existence of conditions without anything more than a definition and a checklist of symptoms. "This is just how witches used to be identified."[6] , he noted.

1. Spiegel, A. The Dictionary of Disorder. *New Yorker*, January 2005, 56–63.
2. Beck, A. T. Reliability of Psychiatric Diagnoses: A Critique of Systematic Studies. *American Journal of Psychiatry*, 119 (1962): 210–16.
3. Rosenhan, David L. On Being Sane in Insane Places. *Science*, 179 (January 1973): 250–58.
4. American Psychiatric Association. *Diagnostic and Statistical Manual of Mental Disorders*, 3rd ed. Washington, DC: American Psychiatric Association, 1980.
5. Hyler, S. E., Williams, J. B., and Spitzer, R. L. Reliability in the DSM-III Field Trials. *Archives of General Psychiatry*, 39 (1982): 1275–78.
6. McHugh, P. *Psychiatry Research Reports*. American Psychiatric Association, Division of Research, Summer 2001.

17. JOHNS HOPKINS DEPARTMENT OF PATHOLOGY, 1949

Rich knew of numerous cases in which the human placenta was infected in tuberculous mothers and readily admitted that infection could easily pass from mother to fetus. But it was in the frequency that he could *find* the disease reaching fetal tissue, limited by the diagnostic capabilities of his time, that Rich would have to speak of TB's transfer from the placenta to the fetus as "rare." William Henry Welch, who besides being a pathologist like Rich was also a bacteriologist, never would have agreed.

Welch was already on record that the mere inability to pick up TB in the fetus or newborn wasn't an argument against frequent transmission to them.[1] There were just too many factors involved, such as the hostile, low-oxygen environment of fetal blood, which could tame even the most virulent TB bacilli into dormant forms for some time, making diagnosis difficult to impossible.

It wasn't only Welch who Rich put himself at odds with. German investigator Baumgarten saw infection of the fetus by the spores of TB coming from the maternal placenta as a common occurrence.[2] In fact, to Baumgarten, who held sway over European thinking for some time, all tuberculosis, including neurotuberculosis, was most commonly acquired in the womb, *in utero*, in most cases— though there remained the possibility that it could occur through infected sperm— albeit a much less significant possibility.

"Welch was already on record that the mere inability to pick up TB in the fetus or newborn wasn't an argument against frequent transmission to them. There were just too many factors involved, such as the hostile, low-oxygen environment of fetal blood, which could tame even the most virulent TB bacilli into dormant forms for

some time, making diagnosis difficult to impossible."

Ophuls mentioned that it was a well-established fact that the semen of tuberculous men contains tubercle bacilli, even in the absence of genital TB.[3] It was obvious, then, that the ovum from which the fetus will develop could also become infected. Kobrinsky cites Sitzenfrey as having "demonstrated the presence of bacilli in the interior of the ovum while still within the Graafian follicle."[4] Friedmann, carefully studying the possibility in rabbits, concluded: "It should be regarded as proved that tubercle bacilli can enter the fertilized egg cell, that the latter does not perish as a result of the invasion, but may develop into a well-formed animal. In addition, the bacilli transmitted in this way may still be present in certain organs of the newborn."[5] And among these organs were obviously the brain and the central nervous system.

That tuberculosis is a sexually transmitted disease is a certainty. By 1972, Rolland wrote *Genital Tuberculosis: A Forgotten Disease?*[6] And in 1979, Gondzik and Jasiewicz showed that, even in the laboratory, genitally infected tubercular male guinea pigs could infect healthy females through their semen by a ratio of one in six or 17 percent.[7] This prompted Gondzik to warn his patients that not only was tuberculosis a sexually transmitted disease but also the necessity of the application of suitable contraceptives, such as condoms, to avoid it. Gondzik and Jasiewicz's statistics are chilling, their findings significant. Even at syphilis's most infectious stage, successful transmission in humans was possible in only 30 percent of contacts. Since Gondzik, many other investigators have confirmed the potential for TB's sexual genitor-urinary transmission.

On the other hand, Schmorl's work supported Baumgarten's and Welch's contention of routine tubercular transmission to the fetus through the placenta. Schmorl's work again showed that, indeed, tuberculous infection of the placenta in tuberculous mothers was much more common than formerly believed.[8]

But perhaps all of this work was upstaged by Leon Charles Albert Calmette at the Institut Pasteur.

1. Welch, W. H. *Papers and Addresses,* Vol. 2: *Bacteriology.* Baltimore: Johns Hopkins University Press, 1920.
2. Baumgarten, P. Ueber die Wege der tuberkulosen Infection. *Zeitschrift. F. klin. Med.,* 6, (1883): 61-77.
3. Ophuls, W. Routes of Infection in Tuberculosis. *California State Journal of Medicine,* 14, no. 7 (July 1916): 272–76.
4. Kobrinsky, S. Pregnancy and Tuberculosis. *Canad. M.A.J.,* 59 (November 1948): 462–64.

5. Friedmann F.F. Experimentelle Beitrage zur Frage kongenitaler Tukerkelbazillenubertragung und kongenitaler Tuberkulose. *Virch. Arch.*, 181 (1905): 150-79.

6. Rolland, R., and Schellekens, L. Genital Tuberculosis: A Forgotten Disease. *Ned Tijdschr Geneeskd*, 116, no. 52 (1972): 2377–78.

7. Gondzik, M., and Jasiewicz, J. Experimental Study on the Possibility of Tuberculosis Transmission by Coitus. *Z Urol Nphrol*, 72, no. 12 (1979): 911–14.

8. Schmorl G Zur Frage der Genese de Lungentuberkulose. *Munch. med. Wochnschr.*, 49, 1379 (1902):1419.

18. INSTITUT PASTEUR, PARIS, FRANCE, FEBRUARY 1933

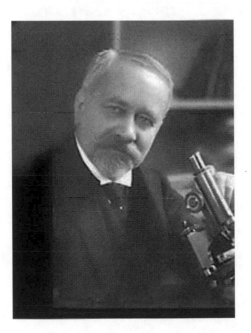

Figure 16. Léon Charles Albert Calmette: Born July 12, 1863 Nice, France - Died October 29, 1933 (aged 70) Paris. Served as Director of the Pasteur Institute. Together with Valtis and Lacomme, concluded

the frequent transmission of tuberculosis, in its stealth filterable forms. from mother to fetus. Calmette also was of the belief that even just an acute febrile episodes from reactivated TB in an expectant mother was capable of breaking down the effective barrier of an otherwise normal placenta. In *JAMA*, Myers supports Calmette, saying "it is possible that a greater number of children are infected before birth than we had ever suspected", and furthermore that "in fact, a considerable number [of such infants] make good recoveries". [Myers JA, Tuberculosis in Childhood *The Journal of the American Medical Association* May, 1927 Vol 88 (19): 1458-60 p. 1458]

"In going against the grain of scientific research such as that done by Pasteur's Leon Charles Albert Calmette, Johns Hopkins Rich, for all his authority and stature regarding the pathogenesis of tuberculosis, was skating on thin ice."

Calmette was on to something.

He had confirmed that TB's attack form going through the virtual filters of the placenta into fetal blood were viral, filter-passing forms of tuberculosis. Such forms were not being picked up by Rich's traditional TB stains or cultures. Nevertheless, they were responsible for wasting and death,[1] even while traversing a perfectly normal placenta.[2]

Koch knew better. Bacteria and mycobacteria certainly could have more than one form. With Almquist, Koch had observed different forms of typhoid in the blood of its victims. Nevertheless, Koch would now begin an intensive campaign to seize and rule the scientific and lay mind that "legitimate" tuberculosis only assumed one form. Thus, Brock points out that, despite the fact that Koch was a first-rate researcher, a keen observer, and an ingenious technical innovator, he went from an "eager amateur" country doctor to "an imperious and authoritarian father figure whose influence on bacteriology and medicine was so strong as to be downright dangerous."[3] And nowhere, according to Brock, was Koch a more dangerous and "opinionated tyrant" than in his rigid insistence on monomorphism, the idea that microbes could assume one truly infectious form and one form only. Yet Klebs, who personally examined Koch's own tubercular cultures, wrote otherwise.[4] In addition to the traditional rods of TB in Koch's culture plates, spherical forms were regularly found, as well as branching, slender filamentous, and granular forms. Many of these could pass a filter and therefore could be interpreted as being 'filterable viruses'. But all of them could revert back and become classical tuberculosis.

Koch's one-form rigidity wasn't making him friends. There was widespread opposition from those who sensed his lack of evidence. They gravitated toward the more realistic, better-documented theories of Nageli and Max von Pettenkofer, which showed that bacteria change forms as they evolve. Nageli and von Pettenkofer's views retained wide support almost to the turn of the twentieth century. Koch reflexively opposed Nageli's ideas as soon as he heard them. Much of Koch's clash with Louis Pasteur was also based on Pasteur's discovery of variability among microbes. In that scuffle, mentions Brock, Koch could at times be so personally vicious as to be shocking.

Vicious or not, by 1939, bacteriologists Vera and Rettger of Yale openly contradicted Koch. Vera:

"The single point on which all investigators have agreed is that the Koch bacillus does not always manifest itself in the classical rod shape. While at times and most commonly the organism appears as a granular rod, coccoid bodies, filaments and clubs are not rare."[5]

To marginalize such thought, Koch and his followers, to this day, have banished all forms, except one, into the wastebasket hinterland of "involutional" or "degenerative" forms of tuberculosis and the mycobacteria. Forms other than TB's classic rod shape didn't count—no matter how many studies showed that all of these forms could regenerate to the classical TB rod, Koch and his minions thus somehow prevailed. To Brock, Koch and his cohorts, up to today, represent a prime instance of the excessive influence of a "cult of personality."

The problem was that someone somewhere down the line would have to pay for such cult-generated ignorance.

Let it be said to their credit that, from the onset, the French saw right through Koch. Tuberculosis had many forms, including a filterable viral-like stage in its growth cycle. Although Fontes[6] was the first to document these, MacJunkin[7], Calmette, and others soon followed. Again and again, either cultures or extracts of organs from tuberculous victims, after thorough filtration through Chamberlain L_2 filters, produced tuberculosis when injected into experimental animals. And, importantly, such forms passed right through the placenta from mother to fetus. In Calmette's eyes, Koch's own postulates were proving him wrong.

Some animals injected with viral, filter-passing TB appeared normal during the time of observation, but when tested with tuberculin showed positive tuberculin skin tests beginning approximately twenty-five days after being injected with tubercular tissue or microbes. Other animals lost weight rapidly. And some died of a rapid progressive infection. It all depended upon the virulence of the strain of filterable TB being used.[8]

In a series of twenty-one infants born to tuberculous women, Calmette, along with Valtis and Lacomme, concluded that their observations proved the frequent transmission of tuberculosis from the mother to the fetus by means of filterable forms of tuberculosis. At the same time, Calmette established that such viral forms of tuberculosis were in the spinal fluid of perinatal meningitis.[9]

It would take time until mainstream microbiology would be forced to even acknowledge such viral forms. It would take a Nobel nominee by the name of Lida Holmes Mattman.

1. Calmette, A., and Valtis, J. Les éléments virulents filtrables du bacille tuberculeux. *Annales de médecine*, 19 (1926): 553–60.
2. Calmette, A., Valtis, J., and Lacomme, M. Transmission Intra-Utérine Du Virus Tuberculeux de la Mère à L'enfant. *Comptes rendus hebdomadaire des séances de l'Académie des Sciences,* Paris. Presse Médicale, 90 (1926):1409.
3. Brock, Thomas D. *Robert Koch: A Life in Medicine and Bacteriology.* Washington, D.C. : ASM Press, 1999.
4. Klebs, E. Weitere Beitrage sur Geechichte der Tuberkulose. *Arch F. Exper. Pathol u. Pharmacie,* 17, no. 1/2 (1883): 1–52.
5. Vera, H. D., and Rettger, L. F. Morphological Variation of the Tubercle Bacillus and Certain Recently Isolated Soil Acid Fasts, with Emphasis on Filterability. *J. Bacteriology,* 39, no. 6 (June 1940): 659–87.

6. Fontes A. Bemerkungen Ueber Die Tuberculoese Infection Und Ihr Virus. *Ann. De l'inst. Oswaldo Cruz,* 2 (1910):141-46.

7. MacJunkin, F. A. Tuberculin Hypersensitiveness in Non-Tuberculous Guinea Pigs Induced by Injections Of Bacillus-Free Filtrates. *Journal of Experimental Medicine.,*33, (May 1921):751-62.

8. Arloing, F., and Dufourt, A. Contribution à L'étude des Forms Filtrantes du Bacille Tuberculeux *Compt. Rend. Soc. De Biol.* Paris. (1925): 165-8.

9. Calmette, A., and Valtis, J. Virulent Filterable Elements of the Tubercle Bacillus. *Ann. Med.,* 19 (1926): 553-560.

19. PATHOLOGY LAB OF ARNOLD RICH, JOHNS HOPKINS, BALTIMORE, 1950

A struggle was going inside the mind of Arnold Rich, and its implications would affect Western medicine for decades to come. Under variations in the forms TB can assume, Rich's words don't always match his conclusions. He conceded that depending upon the type of culture plate that tuberculosis is incubated on, the shape of the organism changes, partly because of the culture medium and partly because of the age of the culture itself. Even the conditions under which this growth occurred, such as temperature and amount of oxygen, figured in. He emphasized that non-acid fast staining rods may be present, especially in young cultures, whereas in older cultures and infected tissues, "beaded forms" were common. Koch also had noticed these beaded forms. Somewhat granular and protruding from stalks, Koch thought they were potential "spores" through which infection could be propagated. But Koch was unable to observe the granules break off into separate segments.

Much, on the other hand, for decades, not only watched the granules break off (Much's granules) but regenerate into classical TB bacilli.[1] Much was also able to document that the granules weren't always "acid-fast" when stained, a hallmark for classical TB which resisted decolorization by acids during staining. Perhaps this was why Much's granules were not recognized as the spores of tuberculosis that would, with time, again become the acid-fast staining TB bacilli microbiologists looked for.

Then there was M. C. Kahn's work. Kahn, using ideal technique, described, in the most precise manner, his direct observations of the growth of minute filter-passing granular forms of TB into fully developed and virulent bacilli, capable of independent proliferation and producing progressive tuberculosis.[2]

Whether granular or otherwise, such viral-like or cell-wall-deficient (CWD) forms of tuberculosis, often mistaken for mycoplasma, are today widely known as "L-forms", named after the Lister Institute by one of its scientists, Emmy Klieneberger.[3] L-forms are cell-wall-deficient by virtue of a breech in their cell wall that allows them the plasticity to assume other forms, including granular forms. Little recognized in Rich's time, L-forms of tuberculosis have since even been found in breast milk.[4]

Rich, working in the 1940s, wanted to believe very much in these viral forms of tuberculosis. They explained the many times that he knew he was dealing with tuberculosis but could not, even as a pathologist, see the germ. Nevertheless, this knowledge, relatively new at the time, was not substantiated enough. After all, Kahn had observed the transformation of granular forms to mature bacilli *in vitro* in a culture plate. This did not mean to Rich that every TB bacilli once in humans had to go through this same cycle in its reproduction. So, despite Kahn directly assuring him by personal communiqué that he had solidified his findings *in vivo* in laboratory animals, Rich was not ready to acknowledge granular viral cell-deficient forms of tuberculosis, which were key to the mystery of how certain forms of TB sieved through the placenta's chorionic villi into the fetus, escaping detection.

Rich's statement that, in certain cases, even when the maternal placenta was laced with TB bacilli, "acid-fast stains of a large number of sections of the fetal tissues failed to disclose a single bacillus" was correct. Welch had predicted it. The viral cell-wall-deficient (CWD) forms could only be picked up by special stains, cultures, and techniques that Rich had no access to.

In the meantime, Rich's hypothetical statement of "rare" transmission was having difficulty. Many infants were reacting to the TB skin test weeks to months after birth, even without known exposure after birth.

"Rich's hypothetical statement of "rare" transmission was having difficulty. Many infants were reacting to the TB skin test weeks to months after birth, even without known exposure after birth."

1. Much, H.   Uber Die Granuläre, Nach Ziehl Nicht Färbbare Form des Tuberkulosevirus.   *Beit. Z. Klin. Tuberk.*, edition 8, no. 85 (1907): 85-97.
2. Kahn, M. C. The Developmental Cycle of the Tubercle Bacillus as Revealed by Single Cell Cultures. *Am. Rev. Tuberc.*, 20 (1929): 150.
3. Klieneberger-Nobel, E.   Origin, Development and Significance of L-forms in Bacterial Cultures. *J Gen Microbiol*, 3 (1949): 434–42.
4. Garvin, D. F. L Forms Isolated from Infection In *Microbial Protoplass, Spheroplasts and L Forms*, edited by L. B. Guze, 472–83. Baltimore: Williams & Wilkins, 1968.

20. DEPARTMENT OF BIOLOGICAL SCIENCES, WAYNE STATE UNIVERSITY, DETROIT, MICHIGAN, 1982

Ida Holmes Mattman, PhD, had an impressive and well-rounded background. Having earned an MS in virology from the University of Kansas and a PhD in immunology from Yale University, Mattman taught immunology, microbiology, bacteriology, virology, and pathology. She worked for thirty-five years at institutions such as Harvard, the Howard Hughes Institute, Oakland University, and Wayne State University. As both a virologist and a bacteriologist, Mattman was equally at home developing the first complement fixation with bacteria-free virus and doing extensive work on various bacteria. And the fact that she was a virologist added all the more credence to her in-depth studies related to viral-like bacterial L-forms (also called Cell-Wall-Deficient or CWD forms). So unique were her findings that in 1998 Mattman was nominated for the Nobel Prize in medicine. In 2005 she was inducted into the Michigan Women's Hall of Fame.

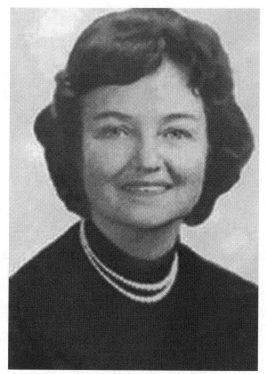

Figure 18. Lida Holmes Mattman [1912–2008] Once the director of laboratories for the United Nations, Mattman joined the faculty at Wayne State University in 1949. She also taught at Harvard University, Howard Hughes Institute and Oakland University. Mattman taught and used a new method to diagnose tuberculosis in 72 hours.

The conventional method takes three to four weeks. Her book, *Cell Wall Deficient Forms: Stealth Pathogens*, Third Edition describes these techniques, using methods widely used abroad. By 2001 Mattman concluded that "there is little doubt that the minute filterable forms of bacteria move from the mother's capillaries to those of the fetus." But what really troubled her, in the case of tuberculosis were those cases, established in the 1970's which reaffirmed that even healthy mothers, with no symptoms were able to pass to their infants cell-wall-deficient forms of TB which nevertheless could kill or injure them. So "stealth" were these particular forms of TB that it once took Mattman eight animal passages before isolating the tubercular pathogen from the menstrual blood of a mother who's infant had become ill a few days after birth.

Mattman authored the book *Cell Wall Deficient Forms: Stealth Pathogens*, now in its third edition. The book is described as follows: *Numerous infectious diseases are described as idiopathic, meaning that "the cause is a complete mystery." For many idiopathic diseases, the causes become clear when certain techniques are applied to the patient's blood or other tissues. Cell Wall Deficient Forms: Stealth Pathogens, Third Edition describes these techniques. In the case of tuberculosis, a disease that has recently regained importance because the strains have acquired antibiotic resistance, the book describes a method that is widely used abroad. This method typically renders the diagnosis within 72 hours.*

If the answer to unraveling the mechanism behind autism was an infectious one, Lida Holmes Mattman was who you would want to have investigating it.

Microbiologist and virologist Mattman knew some-thing that few scientists on the planet still truly understand. Bacteria have a life cycle and can assume many forms. She also knew which special stains, cultures, and techniques would have to be used for the best chance to detect them. Mattman, of course, had access to modern techniques that her predecessors didn't, including electron microscopy, immunofluorescence, polymerase chain reaction (PCR), and other molecular assessment techniques. These helped, but in the case of tuberculosis, especially cell-wall-deficient tuberculosis, they did not always work. She first wrote *Cell Wall Deficient Forms* in 1974.[1] Instantly, it was held in high regard. The problem was that, at that point, not all micro-biologists were accepting it. By 2001, Mattman had con-cluded, regarding the human placenta, that: "There is little doubt that the minute filterable form of bacteria move from the mother's capillaries to those of the fetus." She was refer-ring, of course, to tiny filterable bacteria either without a cell wall or those having a breach in that cell wall. Mattman was an expert on such forms, and as her book went into its third edition in 2001, she also referred to them as "stealth pathogens," which went beneath the radar of modern labo-ratory diagnostics.[2] Once a pathogen like tuberculosis had its cell wall disrupted, it become plastic, having the ability to assume many forms. Some were so tiny that they passed through a 22-µm filter, the so-called viral stage of a bacteria. Cell wall disruption also changed the way these microbes stained. Cell-wall-deficient tuberculosis did not stain with the same acid-fast stain that classical TB bacilli did.

Actually tuberculosis was one of the first placental infections to be accurately described. Since Lehmann's first report, the subject had come under intense scrutiny. Mattman spent considerable time talking about the transplacental passage of cell-wall-deficient forms of TB to the fetus. She knew that of all the pathogens, tuberculosis and its related mycobacteria relied on their stealth, cell-wall-deficient forms, many of them both dormant and resistant, for their singular survival record inside humans. Thus, she was drawn, early on, to the subject. Her 1970 article remains a classic on such tubercular forms.[3]

"What really troubled Lida Mattman were those cases, established in the early 1970s, in which seemingly healthy mothers, with no symptoms, were able to pass to their infants cell-wall-deficient forms of TB which nevertheless killed or infected

their offspring. So stealth was cell-wall-deficient tuberculosis in the menstrual blood from one mother whose offspring became ill a few days after birth that it took eight animal passages to finally yield the tubercular pathogen."

Calmette, said Mattman, knew that TB must traverse the placenta in its viral stage since the placenta, in most cases, remained intact with no obvious damage. Calmette noted that after such infection with cell-wall-deficient tuberculosis, quick fetal death might occur. Even if the child were born alive, it could result in death through emaciation within one month. Yet there were cases in which the infant suffered no ill effects.[4] These were the infants who were infected but nevertheless vigorous for the time being—until the stealth forms of their dormant tuberculosis could spring back to their classical virulent forms. This dovetails with Kanner's thirty-months-after-birth allowance for the onset of autism.

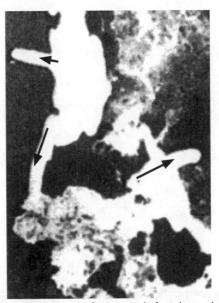

Figure 19. The emergence of a typical, familiar tubercular rods (arrows) from STEALTH pleomorphic (multi-shaped) cell-wall-deficient tubercular growth [Xalabarder, C., *Publ. Instit. Antituberc. Sup.*, 7:1-83, 1970]

What really troubled Lida Mattman were those cases, established in the early 1970s, in which seemingly *healthy* mothers, with no symptoms, were able to pass to their infants cell-wall-deficient forms of TB which nevertheless killed or infected their offspring. So stealth was cell-wall-deficient tuberculosis in the menstrual blood from one mother whose offspring became ill a few days after birth that it took eight animal passages to finally yield the tubercular pathogen.[5]

Mattman warned that tuberculosis mainly grew as ple-omorphic (many-formed) stealth pathogens.[6] In one long series, US labs were only picking up 50 percent of tuber-cular sputum samples by not using special cultures for its cell-wall-deficient forms.[7] Mattman didn't assume that these labs' ability to pick it up in the blood or cerebrospinal fluid would be much better.

Brieger, working at Cambridge University, demon-strated mainly pleomorphic stealth growth when he inoc-ulated tuberculosis directly into the amniotic sac of lab animals.[8] The outer layer of the amniotic sac is part of the placenta. Rapidly, cell-wall-deficient granules formed that did not stain with traditional acid-fast stain. Within three days, other cell-wall-deficient forms such as the long branching fungal filaments of TB appeared. TB is a mycobacteria with both bacterial and fungal (*myco* means fungal) forms. Brieger repeated the study using fowl tuberculosis in chicken embryos. His results were similar.[9] Cell-wall-deficient forms formed, again not identifiable by traditional stains or cultures.

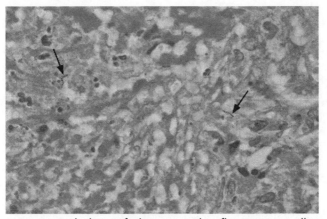

Figure 20. Histopathology of placenta with inflammatory cells and the tiny threadlike violet acid-fast bacilli of *Mycobacterium tuberculosis* (see arrows). Ziehl-Neelsen stain. Courtesy of Centers for Disease Control and Prevention.

While US traditionalists remained skeptical of the clinical significance of Mattman's stealth CWD tubercular forms, the Russians never doubted them.[10, 11, 12] They churned out study after study proving the destructiveness of CWD tuberculosis, which easily penetrated the body's blood-brain barrier into the human central nervous system. By 1996, Insanov[13] warned that an infection with cell-wall-deficient forms of TB in children not only made standard treatment less effective but created a disease with a gradual, insidious onset and a slow accumulation of cerebral damage in children. This made the disease more difficult to diagnose, because its slow burn into young nervous systems allowed months to years before its full spectrum of damage was obvious. Insanov showed that cell-wall-deficient forms in tuberculosis meningitis accounted for an incredible 87.6 percent of the tuberculosis found in children with TB meningitis and 87.3 percent of those in adults. How could such statistics be ignored?

"While US traditionalists remained skeptical of the clinical significance of Mattman's stealth CWD tubercular forms, the Russians never doubted them."

It's not that Americans hesitated to acknowledge the importance of latent or dormant tuberculosis and how it could persist within a child or adult for years without causing disease.[14] They just couldn't seem to correlate the phenomena with Mattman's stealth pathogens.

To Lida Holmes Mattman, it was bad enough that most twenty-first-century bacteriologists still ignored those cell-wall-deficient bacterial forms responsible for much adult illness of "unknown" cause. But with such stubbornness, perhaps, there was a just retribution involved in that the same researchers who ignored her findings were suffering along with the general population. But when it came to innocent children and newborns not being diagnosed or treated properly for disease because of such stubborn recalcitrance, that is where she drew the line.

1. Mattman, L. H. *Cell Wall Deficient Forms.* Cleveland, OH: CRC Press, 1974.
2. Mattman, L. H. *Cell Wall Deficient Forms: Stealth Pathogens,* 3rd ed. Boca Raton, FL: CRC Press, 2001.
3. Mattman, L. H. Cell Wall Deficient Forms of Mycobacteria. *Annals of the New York Academy of Sciences,* 174 (1970): 852–61.
4. Calmette, A., Valtis, J., and Lacomme, A. Nouvelles recherches expérimentales sur l'ultravirus tuberculeux. *C.R. Acad. Sci.,* 186 (1928): 1778–81.
5. *Ibid.,* Mattman, L.H. *Cell Wall Deficient Forms.* Cleveland, OH: CRC Press, 1974, p. 70.
6. *Ibid.,* Mattman, L.H. *Cell Wall Deficient Forms: Stealth Pathogens, 3*rd *ed.* Boca Raton FL: CRC Press, 2001, p. 189.
7. Pollock, H. M., and Wieman, E. F. Smear Results in the Diagnosis of Mycobacterioses Using Blue Light Fluorescence Microscopy. *J. Clin. Microbiol.,* 5 (1977): 329–31.
8. Brieger, E. M. The Host Parasite Relationship in Tuberculous Infection. *Tubercle,* 30 (1949): 242–53.

9. Brieger, E. M., and Glauert, A. M. A Phase-Contrast Study of Reproduction in Mycelial Strains of Avian Tubercle Bacilli. *J. Gen. Microbiol., 7* (1952): 287–94.

10. Gadzhiev, G. S. Characteristics of the Mycobacteria in Children with Tuberculous Meningitis. *Probl Tuberk.,* 11 (1990): 8–10.

11. Golanov, V. S., and Andreev, L. P. Characteristics of Bacterial Discharge in Patients with Different Forms of Pulmonary Tuberculosis. *Probl Tuberk, 5* (1994): 43–45.

12. Dorozhkova, I.R., Deshkekina, M.F., Ereneeva, A.S., Zemskova, Z.S., Ilyiash, N.I. and Zhukova, E.K. Congenital Tuberculosis. *Probl Tuberk., 50,* no. 10 (1972): 80-83.

13. Insanov, A. B., and Gadzhiev, F. S. Comparative Analysis of the Results of Spinal Fluid Microbiological Study in Children and Adults Who Suffered from Tuberculous Meningitis. *Probl tuberk., 5* (1996): 25–28.

14. Parrish, N. M., and Dick, J. D. Mechanisms of Latency in Mycobacterium Tuberculosis. *Trends Microbial, 6,* no. 3 (1998): 107–12.

CONCLUSION

The consensus that autism is caused by intrauterine infection has been growing. In a 2007 issue of *Science,* Patterson hypothesized that by far the most important environmental risks for autism and schizophrenia consist of intrauterine infection before birth.[1] Fatemi, in 2009, mentions the same: that based on major agreement and several decades of studies, maternal infection is responsible, leading toward autism and schizophrenia.[2] The evidence for mental illness, including autism and schizophrenia, being the result of an infectious disease is quite extensive.

Medical residents are often told, "Don't look for zebras. Don't look for the exotic or the esoteric cause of a disease." And the best diagnosticians follow this advice. For the purposes of this document, part of not looking for zebras includes asking what infectious process statistically most affects not only women of childbearing age but their children—and at the same time is nerve-seeking (neurotropic) and fully capable of delivering the myriad symptoms now acknowledged to be the autistic spectrum. According to statistics such as those that can be obtained from the World Health Organization and a host of other sources, that disease, hands down, is tuberculosis and its related mycobacteria.

Just as appropriate, were this the case, might be the admonishment of a resident who brings up the issue of vaccines or their ingredients as a direct (as opposed to an indirect) influence on autism. One must always distinguish primary cause from aggravating circumstance. First, most of the vaccines in today's infant/maternal schedules have a direct contraindication to such potential chronic, even dormant, tubercular infection. And on top of this, physician and researcher Hartz, after sizable human trials, published an article in the *Journal of the American Medical Association* insisting that mercury compounds were "positively injurious and detrimental to one afflicted with tuberculosis."[3] If this is so, then it easily follows that a mercury-bearing substance like thimerosal would only worsen an existing infection. In addition, some of the oil adjuvants used to increase a vaccine's potency are lipids or oils that are cholesterol precursors, becoming cholesterol in the body.[4] Such a cholesterol surge is a big boost for any dormant systemic tuberculosis already in the body, whose very ability to maintain infection is linked to its ability to acquire and utilize cholesterol. So crucial is this unique ability of TB to use cholesterol in the body for both carbon and energy sources that if it were not for its ability to grow off of cholesterol, tuberculosis, unlike other pathogens, would be unable to resist eradication through cytokine attack and the attempts of certain activated white blood cells called macrophages to starve it of essential nutrients. Cholesterol utilization is one of many true survival mechanisms acquired after eons, which has made TB, from a historic sense, probably the most successful human pathogen on the planet.[5]

So in comparative and simpler terms, one might look at an injection of certain vaccine adjuvants, squalene among them, whether inside or outside of a vaccination, as lighting up chronic foci of tuberculosis like a Christmas tree. This does not mean that vaccinations or mercury per se cause autism, although certainly either is capable of precipitating a child's original autistic event by acting in synergy with the infection behind autism. Thus, they could very well *appear* to be its cause.

J. Langdon Down, who was the first to deal with autism in his own children, thought that autism, "for the most part," originated from TB in children's parents. He was also the first to use the term *developmentally disabled* for such cases, a euphemism that the public liked and could much more readily handle than the developmentally disabled from tuberculosis. Was John Langdon Down just pulling from an imaginary short list when he focused on the fact that, in most cases, his developmentally disabled children, including those with autism, resulted from parental tuberculosis? Not at all. Down was a high-end product of English science, and what the British lacked in the well-organized and well-financed state-run laboratories of the Germans, they more than made up for in their astute powers of observation. Down was skilled at autopsy, and his studies' results came directly with how many times he found the disease in his children. Down also could, even then, draw on an extensive library of research on the subject which pointed toward the same direction as his thoughts. It was only then, and after compiling compelling statistical evidence, that he came to the conclusion he came to and published his thoughts.

With time, more evidence accrued. Antidepressants, hailed as new breakthrough drugs in the mentally ill, were really discovered as a by-product of the tuberculosis research of the 1950s. Having proven antituberculous activity, they weren't used clinically as antidepressants until the 1960s. The first was imipramine, now called a tricyclic antidepressant. Almost concomitantly came antidepressants known as monoamine oxidase (MAO) inhibitors, also with antitubercular activity. This was only after it was noted that TB patients given MAO inhibitors experienced a state of elation and euphoria where only depression had existed before. No wonder. MAO inhibitions had activity against their infectious disease.

Yet from their onset, results and studies, no matter how much they confirmed TB's role in mental illness, were tainted by a public that wanted to hear none of them. After all, to be diagnosed insane or developmentally disabled and tubercular at the same time were two of the greatest stigmas that could be thrust upon a patient and his or her immediate family. So insanity or mental illness was either given medical labels that few understood or reduced to a "nervous disorder" with TB always that "not me" illness. Rather it was often referred to as a "chest ailment" during which "nervous disorders" often occurred.

In 1997, Adhikari, Pillay, and Pillay were quite straightforward on a subject traditionalists never have admitted to as other than "a rarity."[6] They wrote in "Tuberculosis in the Newborn: An Emerging Problem":

Congenital TB can result from hematogenous [blood] dissemination of M. tuberculosis after maternal mycobacteremia, rupture of a placental tubercle into the fetal circulation, or ingestion of infected amniotic fluid or maternal blood at delivery. The mother might not have symptoms of TB disease, and subclinical maternal genital TB also can result in an infected neonate.

This seems straightforward enough. The fetus can be infected by the mother with TB while still in her womb. The mother might not have symptoms of TB. And it was an "emerging problem." But another emerging problem was happening at about the same time. Autism had begun to skyrocket.

The extent of the diagnostic problem involved in finding cerebral tuberculosis in infants is documented by Rock *et al* in an April 2008 issue of *Clinical Microbiology Reviews*. In this Rock mentions that some pediatric experts recommend that all children under 12 months of age should have a lumbar puncture due to both their susceptibility to cerebral tuberculosis and the difficulty in clinically evaluating infants with it.[7] Most will not entertain this, but it does emphasize the extreme difficulty in diagnosing the disease in infants.

Similarly, by 1999, Pillet, in an article in the *Archives of Pediatrics*, went over the difficulties in early diagnosis of neonatal tuberculosis. His conclusion, and the conclusion of so many others before him, was that its frequency was being underestimated and its diagnosis often difficult because its initial manifestations were often delayed.[8] By stating this, Pillet was saying what Insanov, Calmette and Welch had already brought up regarding the distinct delay of disease process as a result of the cell-wall-deficient forms of tuberculosis in the newborn which would take time to revert to classical disease. This is also what Mattman brought attention to. Calmette warned pathologists that CWD forms caused few tissue changes to the placenta, and Mattman warned that even healthy, otherwise asymptomatic pregnant women with a focus of tuberculosis somewhere in their body could generate stealth, cell-wall-deficient forms of tuberculosis into the blood to infect their fetuses. Rich had already pointed out the extreme activation of even silent TB that occurs during pregnancy, a fact he had acquired from Norris before him.[9]

In October 2003, Gourion[10] and Pelissolo reported in the *Journal of Autism and Developmental Disorders* on how neonatal cerebral tuberculosis had evolved into a member of the autistic spectrum of disorders, namely Asperger's syndrome.

More importantly, Gourion mentions that a cross-comparison between neuropathology and imaging studies done on TB meningoencephalitis (Hosoglu 1998)[11], (Ozates 2000)[12] and those from the autistic spectrum, including Asperger's (Murphy 2002)[13] (Haznedar 2000)[14] (Happe 1996)[15], seemed to match, including a study of the decreased metabolism in the brain's cingulate gyri. This was important.

In linking Asperger's syndrome, a known disease in the autistic spectrum to neonatal TB meningitis Gourion and his colleagues Pélissolo, Orain-Pélissolo and Lepine joined Schoeman's previous implication that tuberculosis and its neonatal brain lesions were behind the neurodevelopmental disorders, including the autistic spectrum of infancy, childhood, and beyond.[16]

No one who has ever witnessed the pathetic head banging of an autistic child can truly come away unswayed. Many explanations have been offered by workers in the field, some of them unconvincing. That pain relief is a possibility has occurred to a few. They mention a child is more likely, for example, to bang his or her head when the child has an ear infection or is suffering from some other physical discomfort in the head. This makes sense, but some of the other explanations do not. Five out of 11 of Kanner's initial subjects, through measurement, "had relatively large heads", which could indicate possible degrees of hydrocephalus. Delacato, evaluating 474 children diagnosed as autistic found 81 percent of these to have enlarged ventricles on computerized tomography[17], a premier radiologic feature of hydrocephalus. Edwards and many others have documented the chronic headaches that can result from hydrocephalus[18], one of whose more frequent causes in infants is perinatal infection. In fact hydrocephalus itself is often listed as a possible cause for autism. As previously mentioned, at one time, the diagnosis of acute hydrocephalus was so commonly associated with cerebral tuberculosis that the terms were used interchangeably.

It is for all of these considerations, as well as for the sake of the developmentally disabled and autistic children in our midst today, no less those that will grow to adolescence and adulthood, that we carefully review the historic and present debate of tuberculosis's stealth role in the psychiatrically impaired and those children that are developmentally disabled or autistic.

1. Patterson, P. H. Maternal Effects on Schizophrenia Risk. *Science*, 318 (2007): 576–77.
2. Fatemi, S. H. Multiple Pathways in Prevention of Immune-Mediated Brain Disorder: Implications for the Prevention of Autism. *J Neuroimmunol*, 217, no. 1–2 (December 10, 2009): 8–9.
3. Hartz, H. J. Ultimate Results in the Treatment of Pulmonary Tuberculosis with Mercury Succinimid. *Journal of the American Medical Association*, 55, no. 11 (September, 1910): 915–18.
4. Carlson, B. C., Jansson, A. M., and Larsson, A. The Endogenous Adjuvant Squalene Can Induce a Chronic

T-Cell-Mediated Arthritis in Rats. *American Journal of Pathology,* 156, no. 6 (June 2000): 2057–65.

5. Pandey, A. K. Sassetti. Mycobacterial Persistence Requires the Utilization of Host Cholesterol. *PNAS,* 105, no. 11 (March 18, 2008): 4376–80.

6. Adhikari, M., Pillay, T., and Pillay, D.G. Tuberculosis in the Newborn: An Emerging Problem. Pediatr Infect Dis, 16 (1997): 1108–12.

7. Rock, R.B., Olin, M., Baker, C.A., Moliter, T.W., Peterson, P.K. Central Nervous System Tuberculosis: Pathogenesis and Clinical Aspects. *Clinical Microbiology Reviews.* 21, no. 2 (April 2008): 243-261.

8. Pillet, P., and Grill, J. Congenital Tuberculosis: Difficulties in Early Diagnosis. *Arch Pediatr,* 6, no. 6 (June 1999): 635–39.

9. Norris, C.C. *Gynecolological and Obstetrical Tuberculosis.* New York .D. Appleton and Company, 1921.

10. Gourion, D., Pélissolo, A., Orain-Pélissolo, S, Lepine JP Neonatal Tuberculous Meningitis in a Patient with Asperger's Syndrome. *Journal of Autism and Developmental Disorders,* 33, no. 5 (October 2003): 559–60.

11. Hosoglu, S., Ayaz, C., Kokoglu, O.F., Ceviz, A. Tuberculous Meningitis in Adults: An Eleven-Year Review.

International Journal of Tubercular Lung Disease, 7 (July 1998): 553-7.

12. Ozates, M., Kemologlu, S., Gürkan, F., Ozcan, U. CT of the Brain in Tuberculous Meningitis. A Review of 289 Patients. *Acta Radiol.* 41, no. 1 (January, 2000): 13-17.

13. Murphy, D.G. Critchley, H.D., Schmitz, N., McAlonan G. Asperger Sydrome: a proton magnetic Resonance Spectroscopy Study of Brain. *Archives of General Psychiatry.* 59, no. 10 (October 2002): 885-91.

14. Haznedar, M.M., Buchsbaum, M.S., Wei T.C. Hof, P.R. Limbic Circuitry in Patients With Autism Spectrum Disorders Studied with Positron Emission Tomography and Magnetic Resonance Imaging. *Amercian Journal of Psychiatry.* 157, no.12 (December 2000): 1994-2001.

15. Happé, F., and Frith, U. The Neuropsychology of Autism. *Brain.* 119, pt. 4 (August 1996): 1377-400.

16. Schoeman, C. J., and Herbst, I. The Effect of Tuberculous Meningitis on the Me and Motor Development of Children. *South African Medical Journal,* 87, no. 1 (1997): 70–72.

17. Delacato, D.F., Szegda, D.T. and Parisi, A. Neurophysiological View of Autism: Review of Recent Research As It Applies to the Delacato Theory of Autism.

Developmental Brain Dysfunction. 7, nos. 2-3 (March-June 1994):129-131.

18. Edwards, J.E., Britz, G.W. and Marsh H. Chronic Headaches Due to Occult Hydrocephalus. 96, no. 2 (February 2003): 77-8.

Lawrence Broxmeyer, MD